UNDER-STANDING YOUR ALLERGY

HERMAN HIRSCHFELD, M.D., F.A.C.A.

ARCO PUBLISHING, INC.
219 Park Avenue South, New York, N.Y. 10003

To all my patients

First Edition, Second Printing, 1980

Published by Arco Publishing, Inc.
219 Park Avenue South, New York, N.Y. 10003

Copyright © 1979 by Arco Publishing, Inc.

Library of Congress Cataloging in Publication Data

Hirschfeld, Herman, 1904–
Understanding your allergy

1. Allergy   I. Title.

RC584.H49   616.9′7   78-20439
ISBN 0-668-04709-7 (Paper Edition)

Printed in the United States of America

CONTENTS

PREFACE

Do you have pets? Do you like flowers? Do you attend the theater or the movies? Do you wear clothes? Do you take medicine? Do you drink beverages such as milk, hot chocolate, coffee, or tea? If so, you are quite likely to find yourself among the two thirds of the population who, in varying degrees, suffer from allergies.

However, despite the fact that tens of millions of Americans suffer from some type of allergy, most of these people go through pain and discomfort because of their ignorance about the nature of allergic disease.

Since allergies manifest themselves in a variety of ways, from asthmatic attacks and hay fever symptoms to hives and the swelling of glands, people often ascribe their allergies to some other cause. Because of this ignorance—of not knowing what exactly an allergy is—they don't realize the extent of its reach, and suffer needlessly. Or, people simply can't believe that it is "only" an allergy; it must be something else.

Recently, a young child with a marked degree of deafness was brought to my office for allergy testing. His family physician couldn't find any physical cause for the child's impairment. Receiving the child's medical history, he had suggested to the parents that the child be tested for a possible allergy. Sure enough, the child was found to be sensitive to certain pollens, and after a few months of treatment his hearing improved.

Such incidents occur quite frequently in the field of allergy. However, the many people I see in my office each day are just as uncomfortable and incapacitated by their less spectacular cases of allergy as was the little boy who couldn't hear.

The superstitions and misconceptions which grow out of ignorance cause further misunderstanding.

For example, years ago, the disease "catarrh" was quite common; in reality, it was the popular name for an allergic condition. Today, catarrh has all but disappeared—in name only, that is. The allergic condition is still very much with us.

In its stead, we now have other popular diseases, such as "rose fever," "hay fever," and "summer cold." Many people do not realize that their symptoms are caused by pollen allergy, and therefore, they may suffer unnecessary discomfort from a condition which can be treated and alleviated.

But even if an individual decides to visit a doctor to treat his allergy, his misconceptions about allergy and its many manifestations may still be with him, making it difficult for his physician to treat him effectively.

Thus, it is important to have a citizenry so well informed about the nature and scope of allergic disease that all the superstitions and old wives' cures still believed in and practiced will be completely abandoned and forgotten.

The purpose of this book, therefore, is to explain in everyday language what allergy is, its various aspects, its causes, methods of treatment, and what to expect from such treatment. To simplify reading, involved intricate explanations, which are purely technical in nature, have been omitted.

Thanks to Ms. S. Philips for her help in the preparation of this book.

Special thanks to Seth M. Hirschfeld, M.D., who provided invaluable editing and research.

PART I

INTRODUCTION

The body has a department of defense

In the infinitely complex chemical plant which comprises the human body, the immune system is the department of defense. It is there to guard us against invading germs and other threats. In the allergic person, overzealous sentries—elements within the body—overreact to "foreigners," often ordinarily harmless substances or conditions. And the body's tissues, unlucky bystanders, are hurt.

Moreover, once so programmed by these sentries, the body reacts in the same way to the same substance or substances whenever they are inhaled, eaten, touched, or injected.

A commonplace word, often misunderstood

Once allergy was considered unimportant by many physicians and was not well understood by

3

them. Today allergy is a commonplace word, no longer confined to a place in the medical dictionary. Like many words, its very popularity causes many misconceptions in the layman's understanding of the condition.

More than a common affliction

Probably more than 35 million Americans suffer from serious or chronic allergies. These may range from the sniffling and sneezing of hay fever, through the wheezing and difficult breathing of asthma, to a dangerous reaction to an insect sting or the injection of a drug. If we count the minor allergies, such as a skin rash from eating a certain type of food, or contact with a certain detergent, dye, or fabric, then the figure would be closer to 100,000,000.

Not for amateur help

One of the most chronic of diseases, allergy affects people from infancy to old age. It may undergo rapid and inexplicable changes. Because it is so complex, it requires more expertise in treatment and more time and study by the physician than most diseases. Fortunately, today, there are better trained physicians in this specialty than ever before.

The more knowledgeable patient gets better results

The substances and conditions that trigger allergic reactions are endless. Many are easily determined by skin testing. Today, a fairly complete allergic workup can be done in one day. But sometimes the underlying cause or causes are obscure and may call for probing into the patient's personal life and environment. Such a patient, or any patient, who understands the nature of his disease and the necessity for his full cooperation with the physician is apt to get superior results from his treatment.

Chapter I
ALLERGY: A BRIEF HISTORY

Sniffle, sneeze, scratch, cough, wheeze. For thousands of years people have been observing others doing these things at certain seasons of the year, after eating certain foods, or even at changes in the weather. Although any real understanding of allergic disease is new, the symptoms are as old as recorded history.

The Chinese, the Egyptians, and the ancient Hebrews noticed

Nearly five thousand years ago, in 3000 B.C., the emperor of China, Shen Nung, decreed that pregnant women should be forbidden chicken, fish, or horsemeat. Apparently, according to the ancient writings, skin sores had been noted after the eating of these foods.

Then, in 2641 B.C., King Menes of Egypt died after

suffering the sting of a hornet. Hieroglyphics tell us that his symptoms were similar to those described in case histories today.

Certain dietary laws in the Old Testament are thought by some scholars to be based on avoiding common allergies to food, or combinations of food.

The Greeks had a word for it

In 450 B.C., Hippocrates, the Father of Medicine, described the symptoms of asthma, a most common allergic disease. Asthma means "panting" in Greek.

In the second century A.D., Galen, another Greek physician, described people who always sneezed when certain plants and flowers were present. Galen was also familiar with migraine headaches.

At long last progress

In comparison to the amount of time during which allergies have plagued man, the years spent in evolving meaningful treatments for them are woefully short. Even in the eighteenth century, cold water shower-baths were typical treatments for hay fever.

We owe our first clinical description of this common allergic reaction to Dr. John Bostock who, on March 16, 1819, read a paper entitled "Case of Periodical Affectations of the Eyes and Chest" before the Royal Medical and Chirurgical Society in London. In this paper, Dr. Bostock gave the history and clinical symptoms of his own hay fever. Nine years later, he gave a more erudite account of his illness and called it "catarrhus aestivus," or "summer catarrh," although since his previous publication, the affliction had come to be popularly known as "hay fever." The German school recognized Bostock's great contribution by calling the condition "Bostock's catarrh." Bostock disagreed with his contemporary, Dr. William Gordon, who advanced the theory that hay fever was caused by the aroma emitted by the flowers of grasses. Dr. Gordon noted in particular that this condition occurred when the grasses first flowered and passed when the flowering was over. Dr. Bostock held firmly to the theory that hay fever was caused by exposure to the sun. Other physicians of the time cloaked their ignorance of what we now call allergic reactions and their causes by diagnosing them as hysteria or neuroses.

More detective work

Further enlightenment on the subject came in 1902 when Dr. Charles Richet, in Paris, announced the discovery of a phenomenon which he called "anaphylaxis." His discovery was based upon the fact that dogs showed no reaction when first injected with a harmless solution of sea "anemone," but often died from a subsequent injection of the same solution. Dr. Richet used the word "anaphylaxis" to mean "removal of protection" as opposed to "prophylaxis" which means "favoring protection."

Later, Dr. Clemens von Pirquet, in 1906, suggested that the term "allergy" was preferable to anaphylaxis because, obviously, one does not need protection against a harmless solution. "Allergy" means "an altered capacity to react," or "altered reactivity." Therefore, it describes the state of being allergic but makes no attempt to explain it. The term "allergen" is applied to any substance which causes an allergic reaction.

More advances

After this basic understanding, progress became much more rapid. In 1909, Dr. H. F. Gilette studied cases of prompt or sudden death after diphtheria antitoxin injections and noted their similarity to anaphylaxis. From these observations and those of other scientists, allergists evolved the theory that patients become sensitized or allergic to any specific substance following their first exposure to it. This reaction is essentially the same as that of the dogs to sea anemone in Dr. Richet's experiments which were previously mentioned.

From 1910 to 1920, great strides were made in the development of standard methods of diagnosis and treatment. This included the discovery of new allergens and the standardization of the use of the patch test.

Further research brought forth, in 1921, the significant Prausnitz-Kustner reaction which demonstrated that the factor which causes a patient to be allergic could be transferred from the serum of allergic patients to nonallergic patients. In 1935, allergists found that after a patient had been injected with pollen extracts, antibodies appeared in the serum of his blood. These antibodies neutralized his reaction to pollen allergens to which he had formerly been sensitive.

Just a few years ago, Dr. Kimishige Ishizaka and his wife, Dr. Teruko Ishizaka, discovered the function of Immunoglobulin E and other antibodies.

Antibodies, allergens, and Immunoglobulin E will be discussed in the next chapter.

Chapter II
CAUSES OF ALLERGY

What about the immune system?

Within the body's department of defense, the immune system, there are two branches that are important factors in the overreaction that is allergy.

In chemical terms, any foreign substance which enters the body is an antigen. Challenged, the body produces an antibody which fits as neatly with the antigen as two pieces of a jigsaw puzzle. This antibody is formed to neutralize the effect of the "foreigner." Then the body keeps a pattern of the antibody on hand in case of further invasion, at which time it can produce antibodies in quantity. The antigen could be a mold, a bacterium, or a virus. But the body may also produce an antibody to fit an ordinarily harmless substance, such as pollen.

Of the antibodies, five classes have been discovered. Of the five, Immunoglobulin E, IgE for

11

short, is the most important factor in allergic reactions.

There is also cellular immunity, another branch of the immune system, which is the important factor in certain skin allergies.

What is an allergen?

An allergen is any antigen that causes an overreaction or sensitive reaction within your body. It may be animal, mineral, or vegetable. The term can be applied to cat dander, a serving of spinach, or a new antibiotic. Any one of these things could make some of you dash for a stack of paper tissues or break out in an ugly rash. There is an endless list, and new ones which affect the allergic individual come to light daily. The list includes everything under the sun, including the sun itself.

What type of person develops allergies?

Virtually anyone may develop an unimportant, mild allergy. The person prone to allergic disease, however, is inclined to have an easily stimulated vagus (parasympathetic) nervous system. This nervous system is a division of the autonomic nervous system which cannot be controlled by the will. For instance, you can't talk yourself into perspiring or not perspiring. When the vagus system is stimulated, the eye muscles contract and become stimulated along with the glands and muscles of the bronchial tubes, stomach, small and large intestines, or colon. Another division of the autonomic nervous system is the sympathetic nervous system. When stimulated, this relaxes these muscles and decreases gland secretions. For good health, there should be a balance between these two divisions of the autonomic nervous system. For the person with the easily stimulated vagus system, however, not only common allergens, but also changes in the weather, fatigue, or another disease can precipitate an attack of allergic disease.

What about your family?

It is well known that certain allergic diseases like asthma, hay fever, and migraine tend to run in families. If both parents have allergies, the chances of a child developing one before the age of ten years is 75 percent. If only one parent has an allergy, then the chances of a child developing an allergy before he is twenty years of age is 50 percent. The more remote the allergy in family history, the later in life the allergy develops.

However, a specific allergy is not transferred from parent to child. Only the ability to react to an allergen is inherited. In one family, for instance, the mother had indigestion whenever she ate lobster. The father had asthma during ragweed season. The son broke out in a rash when he wore wool sweaters. The daughter suffered from hay-fever-like symptoms when she applied a face powder containing orris root. This family history, as well as much other evidence, clearly shows that children do not inherit their parents' allergies.

Although some investigators have doubted this hereditary tendency, recent studies on genes, the hereditary factor, have strengthened former evidence, and today this theory is in good standing.

If all this seems complicated, and it is, just remember that you cannot "catch" an allergy the way you catch a cold.

What about your environment?

The tendencies you inherited from your parents will do everything possible to join forces with whatever allergen is abundant in your community. If you live in a humid city, such as New Orleans, your ability to become allergic can find an outlet by making use of the huge supply of mold allergens present along the seacoast. There, your chances of contracting asthma from mold would be many times greater than in arid Albuquerque.

Suppose you go north. The possibility of escaping sensitization would not improve. In the regions of the Great Lakes and Niagara Falls, there is another prevalent allergen. It is the tiny particles of the skin shed by the caddis fly. From these minute scales, many cases of hay fever and asthma develop every spring.

Travelling west from the Great Lakes, you come to the heavily wooded sections of the Northwest with still another sensitizer. This substance is the pollen given off by the trees in the spring. Here, the forests are things of beauty only to those who do not have to gaze upon them through irritated eyes or over a handkerchief frantically clutched to a running nose.

The number of people who are sent into sniffles by tree pollen is minute when compared to those who react to ragweed. From the time this busy plant starts pollinating in mid-August until the first frost, the air is filled with the sneezing, wheezing, and nose-blowing of millions of Americans from Maine to

California. It is little wonder that these unfortunate persons wait eagerly for the first signs of approaching winter.

Is it all in your head?

Most physicians now agree that allergies are physical reactions, not emotional or psychological disorders. On the other hand, worry and fear can contribute to an asthmatic episode, hives, and other allergic diseases.

Progress exacts a price

Were it not for the great strides of modern science and industry, the number of allergens causing discomfort would be much greater. Almost daily, new substances are added to our lives. All of them are designed to give comfort, lengthen life, or improve our appearance. This aim is realized in the majority of people who use these products. However, there is always a small group of people who are unable to benefit from a new discovery—the allergic.

This is the era of antibiotics, and most bacterial diseases have gone down to defeat. People who once would have been the victims of pneumonia, meningitis, and other diseases are alive today. But also, because of these "wonder drugs," many allergic individuals have become desperately ill. Vitamins, aspirin, and other drugs or components of drugs have all caused reactions in the allergic.

Another example of disease due to modern living is the reaction of some people to new dyes. These substances can make even the cheapest fabric attractive to the eye, but can also cause large unsightly sores on the body of a sensitive person wearing clothes containing these dyes.

In addition to the improvements which can be seen or felt, there are many intangible ones. For example, no building is considered truly modern unless it boasts an air-conditioning system. Such systems make it possible to keep cool in summer and warm in winter. However, they also lower our ability to adjust to sudden changes in temperature, thus sometimes causing us to react unfavorably to bacteria or viruses.

In addition, molds have been known to get into air-conditioning systems and begin plaguing the allergic. Humidifiers, too, are not exempt from the influence of molds.

On the other hand, as manufacturers have become aware of new hazards to the allergic, they have developed new "nonallergenic" products.

It is important, however, not to give up necessary medication just because *you think* you might be allergic to it. Be sure to check carefully with your physician before doing anything of the kind.

Food allergens

These allergens cause reactions anywhere in the body, depending on where a person's characteristic "shock organ" is. If you are only mildly allergic, you may be unable to identify the guilty food. The amount of discomfort felt by persons who have a food allergy varies immensely. The symptoms range from mild dyspepsia to extreme nausea, rashes, eczema, asthma, and even suffocation and death. Another group of reactions is very misleading and dangerous because, unfortunately, its identical symptoms make the food allergy appear to be an ulcer, gallbladder disturbance, heart trouble, or a syphilitic rash.

Contrary to popular opinion, the particular food that sets a stomach to rumbling or a skin to itching may be one that has been eaten safely over a period of years. When this happens, it is a sign that the allergy has been growing slowly for some time. It is a very simple matter to set off your "glacier." Merely overeat the food in question. In no time at all, you will be reaching for an antacid. Indeed, the three predominant causes of food allergy are overeating, heredity, and stomach disturbances.

An excellent example of how overfeeding helps to bring out an allergy is shown in the case of George M. George had been severely ill with an intestinal disorder. During his illness, his diet consisted almost wholly of milk. Shortly after his recovery, he found that every time milk was included with his meals, it made him very nauseous.

Another case which would be puzzling to a person who had no medical background is that of Joseph B. Immediately following a dangerous operation, Joseph was given many infusions of glucose. Later, when he returned home, he became extremely allergic to corn. With the thoroughness of a fiction detective, the allergist traced Joseph's sensitivity back to the infusions. The glucose used had been made from corn sugar.

One of the most common food allergens is eggs. They frequently cause indigestion and nausea the first time they are eaten. Some people are so sensitized to eggs that merely handling egg shells will bring on a skin rash. Next to eggs, the foods which usually cause allergic symptoms are wheat, milk, butter, cheese, and potatoes—all basic and common foods. It is not unusual for one person to react to two or three foods in this group, causing a real problem.

Nevertheless, the versatile soybean is a fine substitute for many of these foods. And meats, fish, and other vegetables can add variety as well as ample nutrition to the diet of the person with these multiple food allergies.

Today, when there are more than three thousand food additives used in prepared foods, the problem of pinpointing food allergies is more complicated than it once was. And reading all the fine print on every package and can of prepared food becomes more important.

Airborne allergens

Associated with the vital function of breathing is the most common of sensitizers, pollen. Given off by plants, it is carried for miles by the wind. But not every pollen causes allergies. Before it can do this, it must be light enough to be carried by the wind, must be available in large amounts, and must be widely scattered.

Beautiful plants and flowers attract insects that carry on the act of pollination for them. They do not need any further help in order to multiply. Therefore, the plants and flowers which are drab and unable to attract insects must call upon the wind for aid. In the opinion of patients with hay fever or asthma, the wind does too good a job. It can easily carry the grains of pollen from fifty to one hundred miles. As a result, a lovely health resort in the mountains will suddenly become infested with the allergens—to the great embarrassment of the management and to the disgust of the guests.

Because of the huge number of people who suffer from pollen allergy, there are now daily reports on the kind and amount of pollen in the air—radio stations in the larger cities, such as New York, Boston, and Chicago, include pollen counts in their regularly scheduled weather broadcasts.

If one were to ask, "When is the season for pollen?" the answer would be, "spring, summer, fall, and winter." It is not a question of which season but rather of which pollen. Tree pollen fills the air in the spring. In the summer, we must contend with the pollen of the grasses. From late summer until the first frost, the pollen of ragweed and other weeds is everywhere. During the months of December and January, there are symptoms caused by pollen of cedar and fir trees. Pollens are great for the flowers, the plants, and the trees!

Although airborne allergens are capable of causing skin rashes, they more often attack other parts of the body. Their choice targets are the linings of the nose, throat, bronchial tubes, lungs, and eyes.

Another airborne allergen is house dust, which causes asthma and hay fever. The term "house dust" can mean almost anything. If you were to look at particles of dust under a microscope, you would see tiny shreds of clothing, bits of wood, minute pieces of metal, and hair from the cat or dog. Any one of these substances could cause allergic symptoms and does.

An interesting example of allergy to house dust is the case of James N. James was a perfectly healthy boy in his own home. When he was taken to visit friends of his parents, he always began to sneeze violently. His eyes and nose became red and watered constantly. When he returned home, he recovered immediately. After careful examination, it was found that this strange case of "visiting hay fever" resulted from playing with dusty toys given him by his adult hosts.

Still another member of the group of sensitizers which we breathe is mold. Like pollen, the spores of mold are very light. They are carried long distances by the wind. These spores are borne in rust, mildew, and smut on plants. When they take to the air, their targets, also, are the linings of the nose and lungs where they cause hay fever and asthma.

More allergens from the furred, feathered, or winged

Your lovable puppy can give you hay fever, asthma, or a rash just as easily as it brings you fun, affection, and companionship. So may kittens, horses, rabbits, monkeys, parrots, and canaries.

The allergen from pets that affects us is called "animal dander." This substance is made up of two things. One is the saliva the animal has licked onto his hair, which dries and scales off. The second is the scales which come off the skin of the animal.

Although allergy to furred animals is the type most often found, there are cases caused by nearly all insects, from butterflies to bedbugs. People who react to animal dander have the doubtful privilege of boasting that theirs is a very unique allergy. It is not uncommon for a person to be allergic to Siamese cats but not to Persian cats, or to a collie but not to a terrier. In other words, the symptoms in these cases are caused by only one breed of the animal.

Another animal-kingdom allergy is sensitivity to goose feathers used in pillows and cushions. Skin rashes and asthma are the result. In such cases, the feathers should be replaced with foam rubber, dacron, or other nonallergenic materials.

Even though dogs, cats, and horses are certainly not airborne, their scales and dried saliva are. Animal dander is an airborne allergen.

When touch is the thing

Almost everyone knows what poison ivy looks like and how a case feels. But there's an increasing number of skin allergies caused by contact— something put on the skin—that are less familiar. Men who are allergic to certain after-shave lotions, talcums, shaving creams, and hair dressings know it. So do women who react to a particular face powder, rouge, powder base, night cream, lipstick, or nail polish. All of these products are used daily by millions of people. Any one of them is capable of producing skin ailments. The number of cases of allergy to cosmetics as compared with the number of persons using them is small. Unfortunately, that number is increasing. The ingredients in these preparations which cause symptoms include perfumes, dyes, lanolin, and cottonseed oil.

It is very hard to find out which of the ingredients is guilty because the manufacturers of cosmetics guard their formulas very closely. However, by making certain tests with a suspected product, we can soon tell whether or not it produces the allergy.

Doctors who have devoted their lives to the study of allergy have proven beyond doubt that, in some patients, cosmetics are the sole cause of asthma, hay fever, and severe skin ailments. Despite this fact, you don't have to stop using lipstick because you react to a particular brand. Instead, you should find another brand which does not contain your allergen. Jewelry, coins, soaps, fabrics, rubber, and detergents are all substances that come in contact with the skin and cause woe to the sensitive, or sensitized.

Certain bacteria-killing ingredients in soaps or detergents leave an invisible film on the skin. Some people who use these regularly may show an allergic reaction on the skin when they get out in the sun. This is called photosensitivity.

Allergy to infectious agents such as bacteria or viruses

This is one of the most difficult of allergies to discover because it is so closely entwined with many other diseases. Allergy to bacteria creeps up after your body has been the victim of another ailment. Suppose you had boils or inflammation of the sinuses, or perhaps an abscessed tooth. If these ailments are not treated, before long you may find that you have a bad case of asthma or eczema, and twice the discomfort. For this reason, any infection must be treated at once.

Recently, investigators have found that the initial attack of allergic symptoms may be started by a respiratory infection caused by a virus.

To dye or not to dye?

Today nearly all hair dyes have very specific directions enclosed for the possible user to carry out his or her own patch test to see if he or she is sensitive to the dye.

These tests are important because scaly sores, rash, itching skin, hay fever, asthma, and red, running eyes have all been caused by various types of dye. Dyes in cosmetics, clothing, shoe polish—even in the comic sections in the newspaper—have all caused trouble for some.

A common type of allergy to dye is characterized by reaction to one color only. Anna K. is an excellent example. She broke out in an ugly, scaly rash every time brown dresses, brown shoes, or brown furniture touched her skin.

Another type reacts only to a particular product. This is demonstrated by the woman who suffers from asthma when she has her hair dyed with a certain preparation. Hair coloring not only affects the person who uses it but also the beauty operators who handle it.

The typical allergy to dyes will cause symptoms on the skin more than on any other part of the body. These diseases may be centered on the area where the dye touches the skin or they may be spread over the entire body. As a rule, the rash or eczema will appear only where the dress or suit touches the body.

Whatever the color or kind of dye that causes an allergy, the following conditions determine the intensity and severity of the allergy—(1) the amount one perspires. The person who sweats a great deal will have a more serious skin condition if his reaction is caused by skin sensitivity to clothing. (2) The occupation of the individual. A beauty operator who handles a dye continuously is more likely to become allergic to it than a client who comes in contact with the dye only occasionally. (3) The amount of friction or rubbing against the skin with a dye.

Physical allergens

Let us suppose that you have a pain in your back. To ease the discomfort, you apply a heating pad. In a few minutes, you may break out with a rash and your skin may swell. This is a typical case of allergy to heat. Staying in the sun for a few minutes or becoming chilled on a winter day may evoke the same reaction.

If you are extremely allergic to heat, cold, or light, a short sunbath, a walk in the snow, or a hot shower can make you faint or lose consciousness. Therefore, you should take every precaution to avoid the physical allergen that causes your particular allergy. You must wear clothes that protect your body and be treated at once. This disease is not incurable when handled by an allergist.

Chapter III

ALLERGIES AND THEIR EFFECTS

How fast is the reaction to allergens?

The amount of time it takes for an allergic person to react to pollen, to strawberries, to drugs, or to dyes is almost as variable and unpredictable as the weather. Nevertheless, there are roughly three speeds of reaction.

The first is quick—so quick in fact that the lips, tongue, and throat may swell rapidly enough to prevent the food from being swallowed. This is true in highly allergic cases. Those with milder allergies can swallow the food but soon after exhibit symptoms of pain and vomiting. Because of the sudden onset of the symptoms, the guilty food can be easily identified.

The second type of reaction makes it harder to pick out the allergen. With this reaction, you may eat an allergic substance and feel fine for an hour or so before your allergy overtakes you.

The third type of reaction is even more tardy in appearing. It may be twelve hours, twenty-four hours, or even longer before you notice any symptoms. In these cases, skin rashes are frequent.

The same holds true for pollen, drugs, and dyes.

What happens to the untreated allergy?

This seems like a silly question. Of course, it gets worse. Yet a man who wouldn't dream of feeding his automobile the wrong type of oil may ignore treatment of his allergy and keep on eating the rye bread that gives him a skin rash. But, untreated, a mild skin rash grows into ugly, scabby sores. Untreated, difficult breathing may develop into violent, wracking attacks of asthma. Untreated hay fever may lead to sinus infections as well as to nasal polyps—grape-like growths inside the nose.

The infinitely complex chemical plant that is the human body deserves complete respect and care by highly trained physicians.

Where is an allergy triggered?

Anywhere. But there are differences depending upon the type of allergen, how the allergen enters the body, and where the greatest amounts of allergen-reactive IgE are located in the body. Certain areas may be designated allergic "zones" or "shock organs."

This means that three allergic people can eat the same food, say strawberries. The first will have

asthma, the second, headache, the third, nausea—
each a different reaction in a different zone. Jon K.
had a case of hives from breathing animal dander,
but Lucy T. gets them every time she eats shrimp.
Here the zone and reaction are the same, but the
allergens differ not only in kind but also in the way
they enter the body.

Just as detectives use clues to lead them to a
particular district in a city when tracking down a
criminal, so do physicians use symptoms to lead
them to a definite zone of the body when seeking an
allergen.

Zone one and asthma

Mr. W. reports to our doctor-detective that on
March 4 he had an attack of sneezing, wheezing,
and coughing, and experienced great difficulty in
breathing. These symptoms are all characteristic of
bronchial asthma. Since asthma involves the lungs,
we are in zone one.

In this area, two classes of allergens trigger
asthma. The first is made up of foods, drugs, and
pollens. Illnesses from the second class, infectious
agents, cause more illnesses than those from the
first. These agents are bacterial, viral, or parasitic.

There are different effects from the two groups of
allergens. Asthma caused by the first group—food,
drugs, and pollen—appears and disappears quickly.
Or it may appear in a definite season. It is called
noninfective asthma, and the first group of allergens
is called the noninfectious group.

Asthma caused by the infectious groups arrives
more slowly, is more severe, and disappears more
slowly.

Within this same zone, allergic bronchitis, often a

childhood disease, may occur. In bronchiectasis, a condition in which the bronchial tubes are dilated, there is also often an allergic factor.

Zone two and hay fever or allergic rhinitis

Allergies which affect the eyes, nose, and throat— zone two—frequently consist of dust, food, animal dander, bacteria, and pollen. Again, the allergens that affect this zone fall into distinct categories. One is seasonal, mostly pollens, and most prevalent in fall when ragweed blooms. Other seasonal allergies may affect us in spring, summer, or winter.

The allergens in the second class are present all year round and attack any time, in any season. House dust is the most common offender.

The first attack of hay fever or allergic rhinitis, causing itching, red and running eyes, running nose, and constant sneezing may be mild. Repeated ones become more intense. Three out of ten cases of hay fever become asthma, causing serious infections in the ears, throat, and nose. It is essential to have hay fever or allergic rhinitis treated promptly and properly by a physician.

Zone three and skin allergy

As in other allergic diseases, the skin is the target for two classes of allergens, one outward and the other inward. When any of these cause itching, scaling and running sores, a red rash, or burning, scaly spots on the skin, neither patient nor doctor has any doubt that the skin is in trouble. But the offending allergen may not be easy to track down.

In the outward class are those many allergens that touch the skin. These may be cosmetics, dyes, chemicals, and many other substances. Occupations often become a hazard because of the things that people handle.

Such allergies, whether poison ivy or contact dermatitis, are of a different type than the IgE type. They come from cell-mediated immunity (CMI), again part of the body's defense system, and involve a T-lymphocyte. This is a white blood cell, a sort of patrolman of tissues in the body. A T-cell can always distinguish a foreign agent, and summons other troops within the body to start fighting whenever one is detected. Once this happens, the T-cell multiplies in case the foreign agent tries again to make contact. Of remarkable help when the agent is a bacterium, the T-lymphocytes overreact when the agent is poison ivy or some chemical in a cosmetic.

The allergens in the inward class do their damage after they get into the human body. They may be food, such as eggs or milk, or they may be swallowed drugs or bacteria, but all cause infections in the body.

The outward, or contact type of allergens tend to affect the parts of the body they touch. The inward type may affect the entire skin surface.

Symptoms of skin allergy vary enormously, from hives to dry crusty sores. There are no set rules.

Zone four—heart and blood vessels

In this zone the heart and blood vessels are the targets for allergens such as aspirin, tobacco, or ragweed. Such allergens may disrupt the functions of the heart and slow the flow of blood through the arteries and veins. Obviously such reactions are violent and more dangerous than other allergies.

To better understand how zone four reacts to allergens, we must imagine that we are inside the human body. The lung and blood vessels are lined with smooth muscle. If an aspirin is swallowed, a cigarette smoked, or grains of ragweed pollen inhaled, the person who is allergic to one or all of these three allergens suffers an allergic reaction. The muscle linings of the blood vessels grow tighter and less blood can flow through them, thus interfering with the nutrition of the parts supplied by these blood vessels.

If an allergy affecting the heart and blood vessels is not treated, the patient may develop hardening of the arteries as well as asthma, lung, or heart trouble. Another danger of this zone is blood clots. After forming in the blood vessels, they break loose and roam through the body. They travel until they settle somewhere—this may be the heart, lungs, or brain— with permanent damage to the body or even death.

Serums or drugs used to prevent infections, such as injections of anti-tetanus or one of the newer drugs, may act as allergens affecting the heart and blood vessels.

Zone five

Here, the stomach is the target for allergens and, from this vantage point, sores in the mouth or swelling in the throat and chest may occur. At the same time the afflicted person may suffer indigestion, vomiting, diarrhea, pain in the abdomen, and ulcers.

Reactions may be rapid or slow. In the case of Helen T., twenty-four hours after she had eaten lobster, sores appeared in her mouth, her stomach was upset, and she felt tired and nervous. Since the symptoms appeared such a long time after Helen ate the offending food, she had no idea what the trouble was, and ate lobster again. Only after being tested by an allergist did Helen find out what the trouble was.

The most frequent causes of digestive allergy are foods, drugs, and bacteria. Among the foods which commonly produce symptoms are milk, eggs, chocolate, fish, pork, and chicken. The guilty drugs include aspirin and other salicylates, antibiotics, vitamins, and many others. The bacteria come from any infection in the body. Any food or drug may be an allergen.

Zone six—the eye

Allergy of the eye may cause extreme discomfort and pain. When the vision is attacked, the pain is intense, the itching is nerve-racking, and a person's activity is seriously restricted. The allergens affecting the eye are divided into two groups. One is internal and the other is external. The internal group consists of foods, medicines, and bacteria. The external group includes pollens, drugs, animal danders, and dyes. Ragweed is high on the list of pollens. Eye washes sometimes contain drugs which cause allergic reactions. The animal danders come from household pets such as dogs and cats, or from toys made of fur. The dyes which might be allergens are found in fabrics, and in cosmetics such as mascara, nail polish, face creams, and eye washes.

The symptoms of eye allergies are swelling, redness, itching, burning, and tearing. These symptoms vary with the intensity of the attack and the allergen involved. Unless the allergy is treated, the reactions will become more severe. The eyes may develop an ulcer, scaly sores on the eyelids, and growths which have a cauliflower appearance. Also, the vision may be permanently impaired.

Zone seven—the nervous system

Any food is capable of bringing on an attack, but milk, eggs, and chocolate are most often responsible. Many drugs are allergens of the nervous system, among them quinine, arsenic, sulfa drugs, anti-tentanus serums, and liver extract.

The symptoms interfere particularly with the senses. Blindness, deafness, convulsions, swelling, dizziness, labored breathing, headache, and paralysis of one or more parts of the body may occur. Epileptic patients may suffer convulsions following the ingestion of a food or a drug to which they are allergic.

Another reaction to this type of allergy causes an arm, a leg, or the entire body to suddenly become paralyzed. In still other cases, the patient faints and lapses into a coma after he or she comes in contact with a specific allergen.

Naturally, the allergist's first problem when he treats a patient for an allergy of the nervous system is to determine which food or drug is the offender. Because the reactions to the allergens are so serious, it is dangerous for the doctor to experiment, except under certain conditions. Therefore, he must rely heavily on the patient's case history. This history will often show that certain allergens are to be suspected. When a group of possible causes are found, they are removed from the diet one at a time and the results observed. The allergist also must make certain that there are no infections or organic disturbances. Furthermore, precautions should be taken to avoid exposure to allergens in the future.

Chapter IV
DETECTING ALLERGIES

How can we discover their identity?

Not all people know that beef or feathers, for instance, can give a person a rash, a cough, a running nose, or asthma. Also, allergists have found that about twenty-five unrelated foods, numerous drugs, pollens, and fabrics can evoke at least one of these symptoms. Thus, we must first find *which* causes *what* and vice versa.

To discover the causes of allergy, medical science has developed a number of tests which vary with the symptoms of the patient. They must be used with the caution only a trained allergist can employ.

Two of these tests are still used in about the same way Blackley employed them in the nineteenth century. This physician was the originator of such tests and experimented with them on his own body. He used them on his nostrils and throat by inhaling various pollens and by placing pollen in his nose, throat, mouth, and in his eyes. He also injected pollen into the skin of his arms and legs.

Physicians today use many of Dr. Blackley's experiments as guides. These experiments have enabled thousands of cases of allergy to be diagnosed with a fair degree of accuracy by present-day doctors.

The "scratch" that doesn't draw blood

If you have frequent stomach distress, migraine headaches, skin rashes, or asthma, the scratch test may be a valuable method of determining the offending allergen.

Anyone who fears this simple test would hesitate no longer if he could see one performed. An area of healthy skin is selected by the physician and cleansed with alcohol. Then a tiny, painless scratch is made with a sterile needle. The scratch is so light that the skin does not bleed. Then, a drop of the suspected allergen is placed on the scratch. The allergen is allowed to stay on the skin for from fifteen to thirty minutes and is then wiped off. As many as one hundred tests may be done at one sitting.

Intradermal means "into your skin"

The intradermal test gets its name from the fact that the allergen is dissolved in liquid and injected into the upper layer of the skin of the arm, forearm, thigh, or back. In an area nearby, a clear liquid, which contains no allergen, is injected. This enables the physician to compare the redness and swelling of the exposed skin with that in which the harmless fluid is injected.

The intradermal test is often used because it gives a quicker reaction. The results may be read in from eight to fifteen minutes after the injection. Like the scratch test, the intradermal test is not painful, but it must be administered with care.

The patch test

If you are allergic to a drug, a plant, or a dress, or have an allergy that is associated with your occupation, a patch test may uncover the source of your troubles. To perform this test, an area of the skin is cleansed with alcohol and a piece of gauze is dipped into the suspected allergen and fastened to the skin with adhesive tape. In cases of allergy to clothing, dyes, and fabrics, a small piece of cloth from the apparel in question is applied directly to the skin and held in place with adhesive tape.

Usually the patch is left on for twenty-four hours, although it may be necessary to leave it on for two or three days. If your allergy is very strong, the patch may have to be removed after a few hours.

What the scratch, intradermal, and patch tests mean

After the necessary time following a test has passed, the physician looks for redness, swelling, and small blisters. If the skin is completely normal, the reading will be O or negative. If there is a mild redness, the reading will be 1+, or slight. An increased degree of swelling, redness, or blisters will be marked 2+, 3+, or 4+, respectively. A zero reading indicates that other allergens must be tested. A 4+ reading shows that the allergy is strong and that the material tested must be avoided by the patient at once.

Gentle—the eye test

If you are one of the many patients who are so strongly allergic that you react violently to a certain allergen, your physician may use an eye test. The reactions to this method are milder than those to the scratch, patch, or intradermal tests, although the readings are quite similar.

To perform the eye test, a drop of the allergen is placed into the inner corner of the eye. Ten to fifteen minutes later, the eye is thoroughly examined. The patient who is allergic to the material used in the test will experience redness, itching, and sneezing. This positive reaction will disappear within one-half to two hours.

The eye tests are extremely helpful in treating patients who are allergic to pollen, feathers, and dust.

The elimination diet

This is an effective method of finding out the cause of food allergy. In one diet, the first week, all meats, eggs, and butter are eliminated; the second week, no alcohol, coffee, tobacco, or spices are permitted; the third week, all fruits and vegetables are taken away.

If, during the first, second, or third week, the symptoms of the allergy disappear, each food in the group that has been removed from the diet is tested separately. By so doing, the exact allergen is found.

Starvation, too

Another method is to starve the patient for 24 to 48 hours. Then, one suspected food is added to the diet every 48 to 72 hours until symptoms such as asthma, nausea, diarrhea, headaches, or skin rashes appear. Then, the tests are repeated, using only the last food added, to find out if it is really the cause of the allergy.

The passive transfer test

This is based on the Prausnitz-Kustner reaction: the injection of blood serum from an allergic person into one who is not allergic. The nonallergic person is then exposed to a suspected allergen. If he reacts to this allergen, it shows that the allergic person will also react to that substance. This is one way to prove that a certain allergen is causing symptoms.

Newer tests—PRIST and RAST—the in vitro method

Patients suffering from allergic disease have total and specific IgE levels that can now be *objectively* monitored and evaluated to determine the presence and type of hypersensitivity.

PRIST, the paper radioimmunosorbent test, measures the total IgE level, the total allergic hypersensitivity of a patient.

Radioactive immunosorbent IgE antibodies are added to a sample of the patient's blood serum and react against the IgE. The amount of radioactivity present in this complex is then measured in a gamma counter. The level of radioactivity reflects the amount of IgE present in the patient's blood.

RAST, the radioallergosorbent test, measures the specific IgE levels—the degree of hypersentivity to a specific allergen. Test results are the basis for diagnosis and treatment of a patient.

A paper disk bonded with thirty or more allergens is treated with a sample of the patient's blood. The allergic patient's blood will contain the specific kind of IgE that reacts with the allergen. This remains on the paper after the disk is washed.

Next the disk is treated with specially prepared radioactive antibodies against IgE "tagged" with a radioactive isotope of iodine. These special antibodies will "label" the IgE spots on the paper and a gamma counter will readily determine their location.

Any allergen spot on the disk that shows radioactivity indicates an allergy. The more allergic the patient is to that particular allergen, the higher the radiation count to indicate the more specific IgE in the patient's blood. Today, computers are making the RAST test faster and more accurate.

PRIST and RAST—excellent diagnostic tools

Unlike the in vivo tests, PRIST and RAST are objective tests, unaffected by "external" factors— any diet or medicine the patient may be on. The skin tests, therefore, cannot register with the accuracy and sensitivity of PRIST and RAST, which are more sensitive at low IgE levels and more accurate at high IgE levels. The in vitro tests very rarely get false positive reactions.

As a result, the in vitro tests are excellent tools for determining whether someone is atopic or non-atopic, and for predicting the possibility of atopic allergic disease in children from one to three years of age.

A non-atopic individual has symptoms that are due to a specific immune response to an antigen whereas an atopic individual has an hereditary condition—an inborn error of metabolism—in which cells, intrinsically "messed up," release mediators on a non-immune basis. (Examples of atopic disease are hay fever and asthma.)

By measuring the total IgE concentration in the patient—high total IgE means the patient will most probably develop an atopic allergic disease in the near future—the doctor can know whether the patient needs atopic or non-atopic treatment.

Alerted to the likelihood of imminent atopic allergic disease in babies, the physician can place the child on a hypoallergenic diet.

Therefore, if there is a positive family history for allergy, it is reasonable to test babies and children in that family for elevated IgE levels even before they are sick.

Also, if a child is having a breathing problem such as wheezing, a high IgE level can distinguish between atopic and non-atopic causation, and therapy, by controlling the principal causative factor early, may prevent chronic pulmonary disease—chronic bronchitis and emphysema—from developing.

RAST is used to determine exactly what antigen is the cause of the patient's symptoms. The doctor can now prescribe specific treatment. For example: for people allergic to bee stings, immunotherapy and venom antigens are indicated.

In many cases, when therapy has been instituted with appropriate antigens, there is an initial increase in total IgE which may persist for weeks or months before decreasing.

Thus, IgE levels are measured for three reasons:

(1) To determine whether the patient is atopic or non-atopic by seeing whether he has high total IgE concentration. (PRIST)

(2) To discover precisely what allergen is the cause of the patient's symptoms. (RAST)

(3) To monitor the patient's response to treatment. Since blood samples can be saved, a doctor can scientifically measure the patient's response to treatment over a period of time and know whether to have him continue, or terminate, treatment. (PRIST and RAST)

Advantages of in vitro vs. in vivo tests

While skin tests are less expensive and offer immediate results—in fifteen to thirty minutes—PRIST and RAST offer the following advantages that in vivo tests are unable to provide:

(1) Convenience. The blood sample can be taken anywhere at any time since in vitro tests are not influeneced by any drugs or diets.

(2) No patient risk. Allergens never come in contact with the patient so there is never any body reaction. As a result, in vitro tests are ideal for patients suffering from sensitive skin or severe skin diseases, patients who cannot be moved, and when testing for potentially hazardous allergens.

(3) Accurate and conclusive results. False positive scores are rare since in vitro tests are

objective tests—they are unaffected by drugs or diets. The doctor can thus avoid unnecessary or inappropriate treatment and can scientifically measure the patient's response to treatment over a period of time.

(4) Not time consuming for patient or physician. All that's required from the patient is a blood sample; he doesn't have to sit in a doctor's office waiting for tests to take effect on him. Once the sample is given, the doctor sends it to a laboratory for testing and evaluation. The test results are returned in a few days to a week.

(5) An ideal diagnostic tool for distinguishing between atopic and non-atopic allergic disease, and predicting atopic disease in children under three.

(6) Indicates the success of immunization treatment.

(7) Can be done even if the patient is under desensitization or drug therapy.

What is your history?

No matter what type of allergy you have, both your case history and environment are extremely important. Many allergic persons use their allergens daily while at work. This is true among beauty operators who handle dyes, chemists and factory workers who come in contact with chemicals, and bakers who are exposed to flour. There have even been cases of architects who suffered skin rashes from handling blueprints.

If your allergy seems to be caused by a substance which you use in your work, many questions arise which must be answered. First, did you have allergic symptoms before you began your present work? Second, are the dyes and other materials that you handle strong enough to irritate normal skin? Third, did the symptoms appear within one week after you began work? Fourth, are other persons who do similar work free from the symptoms you have? If you can answer "yes" to these questions, it is practically certain that your allergy is caused by a substance contacted at your work.

The preceding examples show the importance of knowing the case history and environment of the allergic person. This is but a small part of the necessary information your allergist needs to help you.

Chapter V
BRONCHIAL ASTHMA

The acute attack

Tight, tighter, suffocatingly tight! An invisible being is squeezing the chest. It's getting harder and harder to breathe—especially breathe out. Lying down doesn't seem to help. As the frightened asthma victim struggles for breath, his neck, chest, and stomach muscles knot. He coughs. Useless. After a time he sweats, becomes exhausted, may turn slightly blue. What has happened? How long will this go on?

Any asthmatic subject to acute attacks is all too familiar with these cruel symptoms, and so is his family. Several mechanisms have been at work. There's been an allergic reaction, and the histamine and other chemicals involved in such a reaction have caused his bronchial tubes—the airway in the lungs—to swell. These tubes form a sort of tree, one

45

branch in each lung, and are called the bronchial tree. At the same time, the asthmatic has suffered a bronchospasm, associated with swelling of the bronchial tubes, constricting his airway. Thick mucous has formed, the result of oversecreting mucous cells in the tubes. Air is getting trapped in the tiny air sacs (alveoli) at the ends of the bronchial tree. This is why wheezing is being substituted for ordinary breathing—why it is so hard to breathe out.

But that isn't all. Cilia, microscopic sweepers studding the bronchial tubes, have a job to push bacteria and foreign particles upward into the throat where they are swallowed and eliminated harmlessly. During an attack, the mucous plugs are too much for these hair-like structures to handle and they become immobilized.

Such an attack can go on for hours, for days, or, if unchecked, for weeks.

Aftereffects

Acute asthma attacks leave the victim in a state to invite other attacks. Some of the tiny air sacs may be stretched and damaged. Some of the cilia have been destroyed, so that the sweeping system will work less well. The flow of mucous becomes slower, and bacteria will find good breeding places in stagnant pools deep in the lungs. The asthmatic can become especially susceptible to bronchial infection, and infection invites more asthma.

Mild attacks

Most episodes, however, are relatively mild. They may subside within a few minutes, with or without treatment. Or they may go on.

Attacks can occur at any time, often at night. They may develop slowly over hours or days as well as suddenly. Although between attacks there may be no symptoms, changes in breathing are detectable by tests.

A national loss

Asthma affects at least nine million Americans today and causes a staggering loss in working time and money. In addition, the illness costs the asthmatic many extras, the largest and least useful of these is money spent for "amateur" remedies, said to ease the symptoms. Obviously, whatever triggers the asthma attack must be discovered, and to find it takes the work of a specialist.

Not a simple disease

Although the majority of cases are triggered by allergens which are inhaled, asthma is rarely due to one allergen alone. Also, the disease is usually accompanied by other diseases or reactions. For instance, Mrs. F. starts to breathe heavily whenever she gets near a horse, eats chocolate, or wears jewelry.

One of the most interesting cases of sensitivity to more than one allergen is that of Allen E. He is allergic to tree pollen, pork, and grapes. During the three seasons when the air is free of tree pollen, Mr. E. can eat as much pork and grapes as he likes without suffering any symptoms. When tree pollen is in season, he cannot touch either of these foods without experiencing an attack of asthma.

The additional symptoms accompanying allergies

are most often those involving the eyes and nose, which become red and itchy, and start watering just before an attack begins. The running, redness, and itching last until the asthma leaves. Still other symptoms are skin rashes and an upset stomach.

A few statistics

Two out of ten persons who suffer from asthma have both a family history and an early personal history of allergy. But, in 30 to 40 percent of asthma cases, there had been no previous allergy of the bronchial tubes. Many of these, however, have shown allergies of other zones or "shock" organs. Some have suffered from skin rashes prior to their attacks of asthma. Later in life, these people may develop asthma due to bacterial or viral infection.

In addition to a history of asthma in the family, a person may develop asthma from a childhood disease.

Some external allergens affecting the asthmatic

Pollens given off by grass, trees, and weeds are the most frequent triggers of asthma. House dust is still another source of allergy and one of the most difficult to analyze. In one sample of dust put under the microscope, we may see shreds of linen, wool, silk, and cotton, bits of glue, mold, metal shavings, face powder, and tobacco. Any one of these ingredients can start an asthma attack. Together they create a powerful source of irritation. To make all this even more complicated, recently a microscopic mite, *Dermatophagoides pteronyssinus,* has been found thriving in household dust.

Occupational dusts and inhalants

These sources of asthma have been increasing in the last years. Although grain and castor bean have been well known irritants for a long time, now we can add to the list cotton, flax, hemp, tobacco, detergent enzymes, formaldehyde, isocyanates, certain metals, western red cedar wood, and even fumes from overheated plastics. Furs, not only dust from them, but the dye, too, are an occupational hazard for some. About the only thing all these different substances have in common is that they travel about in the air easily, and are inhaled easily.

An occupation conducive to asthma is farming, where the allergens may be vegetable or animal—not to speak of pollens. In addition, the allergic chemist who handles hundreds of drugs and chemicals can pose another difficult problem to the physician. Occupational allergens affecting a furrier or baker are obviously easier to detect.

For some, animals are best seen on TV

The dander from dogs and cats is light and easily carried up to your nostrils. When the asthmatic begins to sneeze and cough, he may decide to rest. If he lies down on a pillow stuffed with feathers, the trouble may be compounded.

The symptoms of allergy to dogs or cats are much the same as those to dust. Although these animals are among the most common triggers of allergy, a number of others may cause trouble. Among them are monkeys, rabbits, horses, chickens, white mice, and even pet skunks.

It must be remembered, too, that a household pet constantly leaves hair and saliva on household articles.

Good food that's bad

One hundred allergic people could get together and list the foods that they consider "bad," and few of those lists would be alike. No one can pick out a single food, or group of foods, which all allergic people should not eat. Mrs. Jones may love salmon and eat it regularly while Mrs. Smith cannot digest one morsel without becoming asthmatic. True, certain meats, vegetables, and fruits act as allergens more frequently than others, but *any* food may cause an asthma attack.

A few of the foods which act as allergens are eggs, milk, butter, fish, beef, pork, and onions; tomatoes, carrots, grapes, and strawberries. To make this list complete, one would have to include everything eaten by humans from Chile to Alaska.

Powdered grains and beans are responsible for many cases of allergy. Among these grains are rye, wheat, cornmeal, and potato flour. The bean allergens include coffee, soya, cocoa, and vanilla. Other powdered allergens are tea, mustard, cloves, cinnamon, nutmeg, and peanuts.

When asthma is triggered by food, there may be a pain in the abdomen, diarrhea, or constipation. In some instances, there will be a skin rash covering the entire body, which disappears when the asthma does.

Many people, by merely entering a room where a certain food is being cooked, suffer an attack of asthma. Simply inhaling the odor of fish or cabbage being cooked may make them ill.

In others, just touching egg shells, orange rinds, chocolate, fish, beef, pork, almonds, peanuts, tomatoes, celery, garlic, pears, or strawberries has the same effect.

"Unhealthy" days in the city

Whereas farms may pose problems to some asthmatics, cities do the same to others. When the air pollution for the day is above the federal standard for the annual mean, the asthmatic must take care. Common ingredients of polluted air, such as ozone, sulfur dioxide, nitrogen oxide, and cigarette smoke all irritate lung tissue and permit histamine to be released. On "unsatisfactory" or "unhealthy" days, the asthmatic should remain indoors in a clear environment with closed windows. Air-conditioning may be helpful, as are charcoal filters. If the air pollution persists, or worsens, leaving the area should be considered. (See Part II.)

Drugs, chemicals, and some ordinary components

Many, many drugs and chemicals trigger asthma. One of the most common is aspirin (acetylsalicylic acid). Reactions to aspirin grow slowly and steadily over a long period of time. From a slight difficulty in breathing, this allergy may progress in degrees until it reaches the stage where one tablet may cause a fatal loss of consciousness.

One of the biggest problems with aspirin is that it

is included in so many nonprescription drugs for headache, sinusitis, and other discomforts. The asthmatic allergic to aspirin should memorize the word "salicylate" and never buy any drug that contains it, because this is the term often used for aspirin or a close relative. It is especially important for him to *query* his physician before taking any medication whatsoever.

Many other drugs and chemicals also trigger asthma. Vitamin pills, reducing pills, penicillin and other antibiotics, and quinine are among them. Even a touch of a mustard plaster may start some people on a fresh episode.

In addition, components of drugs and ointments are often allergens. One of the worst is flaxseed oil, used in burn ointments as well as in laxatives, cosmetics, and paints. Again, for those allergic to this oil, the most careful precautions must be taken to avoid any contact with it; otherwise it, too, can cause a fatal outcome.

When protection turns against the protected

Immunization against disease has saved the lives of many who would have otherwise died. But some antitoxins are produced by injecting the toxoid into a horse, and obtaining the antitoxin from the horse's blood. Anyone who has a reaction against such an injection has become allergic to the serum and, although this has become increasingly rare, it can be fatal. Serum allergy was the first disease to be known as "allergic." Fortunately, today these preparations have been purified to the extent that they are much safer.

Infection—special enemy of the asthmatic

Childhood diseases can leave a legacy of asthma. And almost any infection can trigger it—from a simple cold to an infected tooth to pneumonia. This type is similar to that caused by ordinary allergens. Bacteria, viruses, and other types of microorganisms all have provided double doses of trouble. For further information on asthma in children, see Chapters IX and X on "Infants' Allergies" and "Childhood Allergies."

Aging and asthma

When the adult reaches middle age, his asthma falls into one of three groups. First, it may occur with an attack of bronchitis or pneumonia. If either of these infections is well treated, the asthma will disappear.

The second type appears in the person who has had a little difficulty in breathing for years before suddenly undergoing a real attack of asthma. Such a patient usually has a history of nose and throat infections.

The third type builds up steadily. From one or two faint symptoms, such as mild wheezing, sneezing, or coughing to that of difficult breathing, the case progresses into chronic attacks of asthma.

You and your case history

The information that your physician gets from your case history is vital in getting an over-all picture of your disease. He will ask you many questions which must be answered truthfully and accurately.

It is important that your doctor know your age. The answer to how old you are is helpful in determining which disease affects you. For example, most cases of allergy among babies and children are due to foods—usually milk. Symptoms due to pollen or dust appear, as a rule, before the age of thirty.

Other questions which must be answered are:

(1) How long have you had your asthma symptoms?

(2) What is the nature of your symptoms?

(3) Are the attacks mild or severe?

(4) Do you suffer during one season, or all year round?

(5) Do your attacks come right after you have been exposed to a possibly suspected allergen, or some time later?

You can help your doctor help you

The more you can cooperate with your doctor the more he will be able to help you.

Often the allergic patient can identify his allergen. An example is Mr. M., who knows positively that he will break out with a rash and have an attack of asthma if he eats shrimp.

Intense likes and dislikes for certain foods should always be reported. It is not unusual to find that a hated food is the cause of a child's allergy. We find the opposite in adults who are unusually fond of eggs, chocolate, or some other food. People sometimes become allergic to their favorite food by eating huge quantities of it.

The violence of your symptoms is another highly

important point for your physician to know. Some patients have such terrific reactions to their allergens that it is too dangerous to perform tests. When aspirin, serums, or flaxseed oil are even faintly suspected, they should be avoided at once to prevent extreme illness. Any reactions to bee and other insect stings should also be carefully reported. If you are a patient who is, or suspects yourself of being allergic to aspirin, be certain to tell your physician how long your symptoms have been present, and the names of any patent medicines you take.

What previous illnesses?

Besides avoiding certain allergy tests, like those for aspirin or flaxseed oil sensitivity, other vital factors must be noted in the case history.

The first of these is previous illnesses. Have you had sinusitis, tonsillitis, or other infections? If so, your asthma may be due to bacteria or swollen tonsils. Have you had a previous allergic disease? If so, the chances of your being allergic at present are even greater. In the past, when many physicians were not so well informed on the subject of allergy, abdominal operations were often performed when the real trouble was a case of food allergy. This situation is not as far-fetched as it sounds. A person who has severe stomach symptoms may easily appear to be suffering from appendicitis or gall stones. A person who has been ill is more likely to become allergic to a food that he eats in large quantities since his resistance to disease is weakened. For example: In debilitating diseases, doctors frequently try to have their patients gain weight by adding foods of high caloric content to their diet.

Thus, many patients become sensitive to an increase in a particular type of food—milk or beer, for example.

Whether you are ill or well, your general eating habits are a valuable guide to your condition. Your physician must know how much alcohol, tea, coffee, chocolate, and milk you drink. He must know how much bread, eggs, and meat you eat. He may ask you to keep a daily record of all the food that you eat, with a description of the symptoms, if any, that show up within 24 hours. The 24-hour period is used because some symptoms are delayed and do not appear until hours after the allergen has been eaten.

How is your environment?

Your answer to that question may be "Excellent"—and wrong. You may associate with fashionable people and live in a fashionable neighborhood and still have a bad environment as far as your allergy is concerned. A "Park Avenue" for allergic patients is a home where there are no dust-catching drapes and rugs, no heavy, overstuffed chairs and divans, and no mattresses, pillows, or cushions filled with goose feathers. No matter how lavish or how inexpensive these furnishings may be, they are not a good environment for people who are allergic to dust or to feathers.

We may go still further and rule out dogs, cats, and birds if you are allergic to animal fur or saliva. Fumes from coal or gas furnaces may produce asthma, too. These may easily be detected and should be removed.

The enrivonmental causes of some allergies are harder to find. The variety is great. They can be moldy awnings, shellac from dresser drawers, rotten doormats, chrysanthemums, incense.

Just about every substance can act as an environmental cause of allergy, so the working environment is as important as the home. So are the city's smog or the country's weeds. Every place on the map provides its own particular allergens.

What about the season?

A huge number of asthmatic people suffer attacks during one particular season. When this happens, the most likely cause is a plant. Asthma in the spring months suggests allergy to tree pollens. Attacks during the summer months make us suspect flower pollens. In the fall, weed pollens are probably responsible. If you live in a damp climate, your physician should investigate molds as well as pollen.

For testing purposes, four groups

The task of finding the exact allergen or allergens causing your discomfort may be enormous. To simplify it, they have been divided into four groups— inhaled substances such as dust, allergens that are eaten, allergens that are injected, and substances which are touched.

The laboratory scientists go through a great deal of trouble to gather the allergen which is to be used in testing. If it is pollen, they gather the pollen carefully to be sure that no other pollen than the one to be used is selected. The same is true of dust or foods. After the allergen is gathered, it is finely ground and mixed with a liquid. This mixture is then used in the tests for allergy.

The test mixtures are filtered and purified before they are used. After this, they are sterilized in a process which removes bacteria.

When the test extracts have been manufactured, actual tests begin. Inhaled allergens are usually tested first. The groups vary with the individual doctor, but the following is an example of the groups selected. One group contains timothy, plantain, ragweed, house dust, rabbit dander, and feathers. Another group includes orris root, cottonseed, tobacco, and dog, horse, and goat hair. The third group consists of flaxseed, silk, cat hair, horse serum, and insecticides.

Tests are then performed with each of the extracts in the first group. If there are no marked reactions to the first group of allergens after 10 to 15 minutes, the second group is tested. Then, the third group is similarly tested.

Foods are tested in much the same manner. Greater care must be used in some cases of food allergy. For example, if you have shown signs of being allergic to egg throughout a long period of time, the test fluid is diluted to prevent untoward reactions.

The following method is widely used: Tested first is the most consumed group of foods—which contains a large amount of protein—such as meats, milk, egg, wheat, rice, rye, oats, chicken, pork, lamb, beef, codfish, halibut, tea, coffee, chocolate, mustard, coconut, and peanuts.

The second series, which contains a lesser amount of protein, includes such fruits and vegetables as oranges, grapefruit, bananas, peaches, prunes, apples, strawberries, onions, potatoes, carrots, celery, cabbage, corn, spinach, cucumber, lima beans, peas, and tomatoes.

In the third series are lemons, apricots, cantaloupes, dates, figs, grapes, pineapple, pears, honeydew melon, lettuce, cauliflower, green peas, parsley, soya beans, sweet potatoes, turnips, pecans, and walnuts.

Remember each of the three series may be varied or rearranged by the individual doctor. There is no set rule for the order or for the kind of food tested.

Again, in testing for allergy to things we touch, a similar method is used. If you are allergic to a typical kind of house dust or material, your physician prepares an extract with which to test you.

After your tests have been completed, you will probably find that you are allergic to several things instead of just one. Should this happen, the physician takes special care in planning your treatment.

More facts the asthmatic's physician needs

Have you any hereditary tendencies to allergy?
What previous illnesses have you suffered
(allergic and nonallergic)?
How long do your attacks of asthma last?
How severe are these attacks?

The above questions are just a few of the salient points which must be discussed to aid your return to health.

This information is supplemented with a thorough physical examination, X-rays, blood, skin, and urine tests, and a basal metabolism. There will also be tests to find out how well the lungs are functioning.

The symptoms of asthma, such as coughing, sneezing, wheezing, expectoration, and labored breathing, are well known. Because of this, many people decide that when one of these symptoms appears, they definitely have asthma. They overlook the fact that tuberculosis, foreign bodies in the throat or lungs, pleurisy, and heart or kidney trouble can cause the same symptoms.

If an examination proves that asthma definitely exists, we must then find the allergen which causes it. An infection in the body makes this task more difficult. Examinations show whether the asthma is caused by bacteria or by an external allergen. Some cases are due to a combination of both.

The easiest way for the physician to find the allergen is to observe the patient closely for any unusual symptoms. After external allergens and organic ailments have been ruled out, the allergist starts searching for an infection. Abnormal body temperature is an indication of infection. It will go up if the teeth, throat, bronchial tubes, or lungs are infected. When the infection is found, it must be treated at once.

The treatment

All treatment of asthma is directed at clearing bronchial tubes so that the patient may resume normal breathing. There are two parts to this. The first is immediate relief of the attack. The second is long-term therapy to prevent or lessen the severity of further episodes.

There are a number of new drugs to prevent asthma attacks and to handle one when it occurs. One called cromolyn sodium acts on the histamine release mechanism to help prevent an episode.

When an attack is beginning, use of a bronchodilator will dilate or widen the air tubes. To stop a severe one, a physician may inject epinephrine. In extremely severe attacks which require hospitalization, oxygen mixed with medication may be employed through a machine. This is called intermittent positive pressure breathing.

An aim is always to get rid of the mucous plugs that block the airway. The asthmatic must drink as much fluid as possible, or breathe in moist air. In severe cases, fluid can be infused into a vein.

The long-term treatment seeks ways to protect the asthmatic against his allergens—once they are detected. He must take every possible measure to avoid them. (See Part II for some helpful hints.) Sometimes his sensitivity can be lessened by injection treatments of small amounts of extracts made from allergens over a period of time.

Any infection—including sinuses and teeth—must be cleared. General exercises as well as special breathing exercises are helpful. A healthful diet with extra vitamins, liver, and iron may be prescribed. A person who has had infectious asthma should avoid sudden changes in climate or exposure to cold.

Results are what count

With carefully employed tests and treatment, most results are excellent. Successful treatment depends on two factors:

(1) The physician's skill in finding which allergens cause the asthma.

(2) The amount of damage done to the body prior to treatment.

In more than 75 percent of all cases, the results are satisfactory if the body is not badly damaged, if the cause is found, and *if the patient cooperates.*

Chapter VI
HAY FEVER

The hardest working pollen factory

One ragweed plant can produce eight billion grains of pollen in a single season. Light, dry, dancing in the breeze, it's small wonder that these tiny grains have been discovered nearly two miles up and as far as four hundred miles out to sea. And it's not surprising either that this fluffy plant is the primary cause of hay fever in the United States. For those whose eyes and nose begin to itch and run in August, ragweed is usually the cause. And the coughing and sneezing may continue through September, until the first frost.

What does hay fever mean?

Hay fever does not mean that this cold-like affliction has to do with hay, except for mold on hay, nor does it always take place in August. It can begin

in April and last until June. It can start in May and
last until July or August. And for some unfortunates,
it may begin any time and last all year round.

The symptoms are swelling and blocking of the
nose, running of the eyes and nose, redness and
swelling of the eyes, and frequent sneezing. Any one
of these symptoms, depending on the severity of the
case, may plague the hay fever victim.

The seasons are guides

The fact that Mr. A. began sneezing in April is not
sufficient evidence to say, flatly, that he is allergic to
oak pollen. However, it is an excellent reason to
suspect the cause to be *one* of the tree pollens which
are in the air during the spring months. The season is
a helpful guide to a group of allergens but not to a
specific allergen. In addition to oak pollen, spring
brings a generous supply of elm, poplar, ash,
sycamore, birch, hickory, beech, maple, elder, and
cedar pollens. Any one of a combination of several of
these allergens may cause hay fever. Therefore, we
use the season to guide us to a group of sensitizers.
From there, we must rely on skin tests to point out the
exact allergen.

For some whose symptoms last from May to July,
we would first suspect the grasses which pollinate at
that time. Because timothy and orchard grasses
produce the greatest amount of pollen, they are likely
suspects. Others in this group are Bermuda, Johnson, sweet vernal, low spear, and June grasses.

In those with symptoms from August to frost,
besides the "everywhere" ragweed pollen, there are
also tumbleweed, marsh elder, hemp, cockleburr, and
thistle to start the sniffling and sneezing.

For those whose symptoms last all year round,

pinpointing the allergen or allergens is more difficult. It may be caused by any of an enormous variety of foods, dusts, animal danders, molds, perfumes, hairsprays, and other household products, as well as infection. Physicians call this type "perennial allergic rhinitis."

Unpredictable

The timing of cases of hay fever varies greatly. We must consider the season of pollination and make allowances for changes in the weather. An unusually warm summer will increase the quantity of pollen. Rainfall is just as helpful to the growth of weeds and grasses as it is to that of corn and wheat. A late frost lengthens the ragweed season. Heat and rain aid in the growth of plants and so increase the pollen supply.

What grows where you live?

It would be a waste of time for an allergist to test a resident of Massachusetts for allergy to Johnson or Bermuda grasses which rarely grow north of Georgia. To test a patient who has never been west of Pennsylvania for tumbleweed sensitivity would be just as useless. But your local allergist knows his pollens just as the local farmer knows his fruits and vegetables. He must!

Fruits, vegetables, insects, and molds

All these are termed seasonal allergens. A mouthful of strawberries may start the sneezing for one person. Or a May fly, particularly the caddis fly, abundant in the Great Lakes region, may trigger another's. Or a moth. Molds affect still another sufferer. Although classified as seasonal, their growth depends on the amount of heat and rainfall in any locality. So it's the climate rather than the season that makes a difference to this type of hay fever victim.

How hay fever progresses

The first symptoms seem mild. The eyes and nose run slightly and sneezing is infrequent. Untreated, the disease progresses. Attacks begin to grip the victim at any time of day or night. Untreated, approximately three out of ten hay fever sufferers develop chronic asthma.

In untreated hay fever, sinusitis, nasal polyps, and earaches are frequent complications, and seasonal hay fever can become perennial allergic rhinitis.

A quick trip to an allergist might save a hay fever sufferer from most or all of these problems.

What the sensible person with hay fever does

In visiting his physician, this person provides a complete case history. In turn, the physician does a complete physical examination. Next, the skin testing begins. This is simplified if the patient can provide clues to his allergen.

The test material must be "adjusted" to the individual case. Mrs. Smith may require five thousand units of an extract, while Mrs. Jones needs only ten units. The strength of the extract must be equal to the intensity of the allergy. A strong solution is necessary to make an accurate test of a weak allergy. A weak solution will work for a strong allergy.

A patient is usually tested for only those allergens with which he comes in contact. There is no hard and fast rule for testing a hay fever victim in the North, South, East, or West. The allergist in each case must be guided by the case history and his own experience.

Science has found that a patient who reacts to one member of a plant species or family will react to all members of that family. To illustrate, if you have hay fever from one common grass, you will react to all of the grasses in that particular plant family. This simplifies the problem of testing.

The most widely used allergen extracts for testing hay fever victims are oak, birch, elm, poplar, hickory, ash, maple, and beech in the tree pollen group; timothy in the grass pollen group; and ragweed, plantain, and sorrel in the weed group. This list does not cover *all* of the cases, and it is often necessary to prepare additional extracts to fit the needs of the individual patient.

Pollen charts and counts—two great aids

The pollen chart is a listing of the most frequent airborne allergens. These are arranged according to the season of the year and the length of time that they pollinate. After studying his patient's case history, the physician compares the period during which the patient's symptoms appear with the pollination periods of the various trees, weeds, and grasses on the pollen chart. When he finds that a

particular pollen is in the air at the same time the hay
fever victim becomes ill, he tests with this pollen
immediately. Very good results have been obtained
by using this method.

Pollen counts show just what kind of pollen is in
the air over a specific region of the country. They also
show which areas are free of pollen. To patients
whose hay fever clings to them unless they avoid a
certain pollen, such information is extremely valuable. Pollen counts also give the physician a chance
to discover whether or not an abundance of a
particular pollen affects or causes his patient's
allergy. Response to treatment closely follows the
pollen count. In other words, Margaret G. will
respond much better to treatment for ragweed
allergy when there is less ragweed pollen in the air.

The actual skin testing

Every skin has a story to tell the physician, and
each case presents an individual problem in testing.

To illustrate the use of the intradermal, or "into the
skin" test, let us take the case of Anna V. The
allergist swabs Anna's arm with alcohol at the test
site. Then, a small amount of the allergen is injected
with a hypodermic needle at this site. Six tests are
made at one time, and are spaced an inch or inch and
a half apart in a horizontal row. After fifteen
minutes, none of the first six tests causes Anna's arm
to itch or become red. This indicates that she is not
allergic to any of the allergens used thus far. An area
an inch and a half below the original tests is cleansed
and another row is made. Still no reactions appear. A
third row is placed below the second. Within thirty
minutes, the spot where the oak pollen has been

injected becomes red and itchy. Tiny "hives" appear—the cause of Anna's hay fever has been found.

Anna V., like many other hay fever victims, reacted to her allergen within fifteen to thirty minutes after the allergen had been injected into her skin. If she had been more highly allergic, the time would have been less.

The tests are not painful to the patient and they are rather simple to perform. They must, however, be read with care. The reactions to these tests are classified as "marked," "moderate," "slight," or "negative." If "marked," the test area will be very red, itching, and swollen. If "moderate," there will be little or no swelling but merely redness and itching. Those tests which are "marked" are definite signs of allergy and must be treated at once. The "moderate" reactions are often evidence that the testing extract should be strengthened and another test made to confirm the initial result.

Sometimes an eye test is used, in which a small amount of the allergen extract is dropped in the corner of the patient's eye. If the patient is allergic to the test extract, his eye will become red and itchy within fifteen minutes. Then a soothing eye drop will be used to make the eye comfortable again.

The plan for treatment of seasonal hay fever

After the physician studies the results, he plans the treatment. He may prescribe an antihistamine to lessen some of the symptoms. This cannot be wholly helpful, however, because it fights only *one* of the troublesome chemicals, histamine, released during an allergic attack. There are others. He may try a corticosteroid, a hormonal medication. This, however, is too powerful for repeated use.

Among adults as well as children, injections with pollen extracts for desensitization are effective. There are three methods, perennial, pre-seasonal, and co-seasonal, which must be repeated yearly.

The most effective method

The perennial type requires a patient to take an injection of the proper extract—say ragweed—every four weeks during the six months of winter. In the spring, a fresh extract is given in smaller quantities. The injections are given every two weeks until the quantity of the winter injections has been reached.

Of the three, this is the most effective method. Fewer doses are needed in the long run, the chances for a permanent cure are greater, and the results are better.

The disadvantage is that many patients become careless and miss their injections, lessening their chance for relief. In addition, some persons are so highly allergic that their bodies will not tolerate even a tiny amount of the substance to which they are allergic.

The pre-seasonal or before-the-season method

In this method, an extract is made of the patient's allergen and is injected at from four- to seven-day intervals. The first injection is mild and the strength of the extract is gradually increased until the pollination season arrives. The injections are continued through the season if the symptoms are lessened.

If the sneezing and wheezing are not helped, the patient is given a weaker solution of the extract or the injections are stopped. It is obvious that no hard or fast rules can be made for the "pre-seasonal" treatment. The physician must rely entirely on the condition and the improvement of the patient to guide him. Ten different hay fever victims may need ten different strengths of pollen extracts.

When other methods are too late

Both the pre-seasonal and perennial types of treatment are impossible when the patient begins treatment shortly before, or during, the pollination season. In cases of this sort, the co-seasonal, or with-the-season method is helpful. Injections of the pollen extract are given every two to four days in gradually increased doses. Because of the patient's late start and the shortness of the season, the most beneficial strength of the extract cannot be reached, and the effectiveness of the treatment is lessened.

Perennial allergic rhinitis

Because this perennial "hay fever" lasts so indefinitely—even for years—it does more damage to the body than the seasonal type. The ears, the throat, and the nose, particularly, may be affected.

In many cases, the discomfort begins when a person who has become allergic to dust, pollen, or a food does not take treatment. An infection in the eyes, ears, nose, or throat follows. And bacteria multiply to the extent that an allergy to them develops. In this way, a mild allergy may grow into a dangerous and uncomfortable disease.

There are, however, many ways in which allergy

to bacteria can develop. Variation in this type of hay fever is not the exception; it is the rule.

When bacteria are the allergens

Your physician must find out whether or not your symptoms are caused by an allergen. After finding out that this is so, he then must pinpoint what it is— bacteria or an external substance. Suppose bacteria are the offenders, and a physical examination shows that you have an infection. This must be cleared at once by antibiotics or by some other means.

Other and outer causes

If no infection is present, the cause is most generally dust or animal dander. The dust may be from the house or from one's occupation. In such an instance, the case history must include where the symptoms are felt, the type of occupation, the material handled on the job, and the type of household furnishings.

Patients who are allergic to animal danders, animal hair, and saliva must answer questions about the number, breed, and species of their household pets and those of their friends. Rugs and clothing made of fur provide other sources of exposure to animal danders.

There are only a few cases of perennial allergic rhinitis caused by food in adults. Avoiding this particular food will bring relief in most cases.

Even fewer cases of allergic rhinitis are caused by things we touch. Some people, however, cannot handle oranges, bananas, eggs, celery, or nuts. The dye in a dress or scarf may cause a woman's eyes and nose to swell. The perfumes and oils in toilet preparations may occasionally cause symptoms.

Allergic rhinitis may also occur from vitamin pills, cold tablets, aspirin, eye drops, and nose drops.

You can help yourself

Fortunately for the person with hay fever, whether his disease be of seasonal, perennial, external, or bacterial type, there are a number of precautions that he can take to improve his condition. These precautions are, of course, in addition to the treatment he receives from his physician. He should avoid smoke-filled rooms, which irritate his eyes and nose. Abstinence from tea, coffee, and other beverages which increase the flow of blood, thereby causing congestion of swollen nasal passages, is of help. He can avoid sudden changes of temperature, drafts, and many irritating chemical fumes. Fatigue and exhaustion interfere with progress in all cases. Swimming will irritate the eyes and nose of the hay fever victim. And, if the patient can afford one, an air-conditioning unit which filters out dust and pollen allergens offers great relief. (See Part II.) Last of all, and by far the most important, is the maintenance of good mental and physical health by correct eating, exercise, and work.

Chapter VII

SKIN ALLERGY

The skin works day and night

The skin, a separate organ, performs many functions which go unnoticed until trouble interferes. The duties of your body covering, which physicians call "integument," are vital to life. When one or more of the skin's functions stop, you become ill.

Your skin excretes waste material and keeps your body at a healthy temperature twenty-four hours a day. It also protects you from injury, gives warning signals of heat, cold, touch, or pain, absorbs external material and immunizes you to outside substances. Understanding the skin's functions of absorption and protection is necessary in discussing skin allergies.

A popular target

Designated as zone three, the skin is prone to both inner and outer causes of allergic skin problems. Any patient can see a skin disease. Its cause is not so easy to detect.

Skin allergies may take the form of hives (urticaria) or eczema (atopic dermatitis), both IgE-type allergic reactions. Whatever way the allergen is taken into the body, it passes into the bloodstream and finds its way to the skin tissue.

Today, however, the most common type of allergic skin irritation is contact dermatitis, caused by an allergen that touches the skin. As already stated, this type of reaction is caused by cell-mediated immunity, or T-cells.

There is much variation in people's sensitivity to skin irritants. Men's skin is less sensitive than women's; dark skin less sensitive than fair. Perspiration helps to sensitize the skin because a moistened chemical may become more irritating. In general, thicker skin is less susceptible to skin irritants than fine. For instance, the fine skin on your eyelids reacts more readily to allergens than the tough skin on your palms.

Hives

Hives, sometimes called nettle rash, appears singly or in clusters as red, swollen, and intensely itchy spots. It may last over a long period of time or appear briefly and disappear immediately after the cause has been removed.

Long a problem to the physician as well as to his patient, hives may be caused by drugs and stimulants, infectious agents, foods, clothing, and, rarely, pollen.

Drugs are considered a common cause. Among them, those often responsible are aspirin, quinine, penicillin streptomycin, sulfa drugs, and laxatives. In addition, injections such as liver and gland extracts, insulin, vitamin preparations, and serums may cause serious reactions in allergic patients.

Of the infectious agents, bacteria are most often responsible. Tonsils, sinuses, gall bladder, kidneys, and lungs all may contain foci of infection. But other infectious agents may act as promoting factors. These are fungi, low forms of plant life; viruses smaller than bacteria, as little as one-fiftieth of a micron in diameter; helminths, worm-like parasitic organisms (sometimes free-living); and protozoa, one-celled animals.

Foods are an important cause of hives. Commonly, these may be eggs, chicken, fish, shellfish, or chocolate. Others are seasonal, such as tomatoes or strawberries. In such cases, the patient who suspects the cause of his trouble can aid the allergist immensely.

In some cases, contact, touching silk, house dust, wool, or other substances may produce hives— sometimes in an area where the allergen has not touched the skin. This is because it has been absorbed into the bloodstream.

Hives may also be caused by heat, light, cold, and sometimes even friction. This form of allergy is perhaps the most difficult to avoid.

There are two types of urticarial reactions involving the same allergen:

Type 1—Mrs. V. eats a bowl of tomato soup. Almost at once the skin over her entire body breaks out and swells. The hives last two days during which time she vomits and suffers pains in her stomach.

Type 2—Mr. R. is also allergic to tomato soup. After he has eaten a bowl of it, he has no immediate symptoms. But, slowly, he notices swelling and hives in isolated parts of his body. In a few days, the symptoms practically disappear. Then, they return, subside, and return again. A single attack lasts for weeks.

Angioedema

Angioedema is essentially the same as urticaria. But urticaria affects the surface of the skin, and angioedema involves the deeper layers. Sometimes it is called giant hives. The same or a similar allergen may be responsible for both. There is usually an hereditary factor in angioedema.

Because this condition can affect the throat or larynx, it is more serious than hives, and demands a physician's immediate attention.

Unlike hives, angioedema develops only after a delayed period. The symptoms appear in a specific part of the body, and there is extreme swelling which lasts as long as a week.

All the facts for your physician

Only from the facts you tell him can your physician limit the allergens—for which he must test you to find out the cause of your hives. Not only your family history and background, but your daily habits and any suspicions regarding possible allergens—all are valuable information in seeking the cause of your hives.

The next steps

Your allergist will examine you carefully for any organic symptoms of infection in the body. Frequently, the removal of a site of infection relieves the symptoms.

After the physical examination come the skin tests. (See Chapter IV, pp.35–38; also see Chapter VI, pp. 68–69.)

Food diary

Using the case history, family history, physical examination, and his wide knowledge of various allergens, the allergist makes a selection of the most probable allergens. The suspected substances are eliminated from the patient's diet for intervals of approximately two weeks. By this method, entire groups of substances can be eliminated at the same time. If the symptoms disappear, each member of the group is then tested separately. The allergy patient keeps a list of the kinds and amounts of foods he eats during these tests. Should any of the symptoms come back at any time, the diet of the past few days is reexamined for a suspected allergen, especially those foods which have not been eaten previously.

For symptoms that are extremely severe, the allergist may prescribe drugs, such as antihistamines, epinephrine, or a steroid. These drugs do not cure; they alleviate the symptoms.

After the physician discovers the allergen, the

patient must avoid it, if possible, and the symptoms will disappear. If, however, it is one that is vital to health, or one that cannot be easily avoided, then injections are used to increase the patient's resistance to sensitivity. These are given in gradually increased strength or quantity at regular intervals.

Allergic eczema or atopic dermatitis

In this condition, the skin is red, irritated, dry, and crusted, and it discharges a colorless fluid. Although the symptoms are on the surface of the body, they are caused by an allergy from within. That is why this disease is called an "intrinsic" or "inward" type of allergic reaction.

The allergens that cause allergic eczema or atopic dermatitis are carried in the blood stream. This automatically lessens the number of allergens to be suspected because they must either be injected in the form of drugs, or ingested in the form of foods. When they are ingested, substances are first swallowed. They then pass through the stomach and into the small intestine. Here the ingested food is absorbed into the blood stream and carried throughout the body. The length of time needed for digestion and absorption varies with each person. For this reason, an adequate period must be allowed so the allergen has sufficient opportunity to make its journey from the mouth to the stomach, small intestine, blood stream, and finally to circulate through the system. Obviously, symptoms will not appear as quickly as when an allergic person touches wool.

The two kinds of allergens most often suspected— and most often found guilty—of causing allergic eczema are foods and drugs. Among the common food allergens are milk, eggs, and wheat. That is why many cases of eczema are found among babies. These substances not only compose a large part of the infant's diet, but are, of course, the first foods they eat.

A number of cases of allergic eczema are caused by drugs, both swallowed and injected. Among these are the sulfa drugs, vitamin and liver extracts, and coal-tar products. Sensitivity to a particular one causes identical symptoms whether the drug is taken by mouth, applied to the skin, or injected. The only difference is that an injection produces a reaction more quickly.

Bacteria from an infection within the body or on its surface also causes eczema if the bacteria gets into the blood stream. In connection with allergic skin conditions from infections, we must not forget the part played by patent medicines. Robert W. is a good example of the unhappy result of self-treatment.

Mr. W. frequently told his friends that he "wasn't the type who ran to the doctor every time he stubbed his toe." While attending a beach party, he cut his foot slightly on a piece of jagged glass. Although there was no infection, he decided to hurry the healing process by applying an ointment of his own choice to the cut. A week later, he noticed patches of weeping eczema on his body. When he was finally persuaded to see a doctor, Robert W. was found to be allergic to a drug in the ointment. Had he received professional treatment at the time his foot was cut, he would have avoided both the discomfort and the expense of eczema.

Fortunately, the number of cases of allergy to substances carried in the blood stream is not as large

as those due to external or outside causes. Because of
this, exceptional care is taken to examine the
patient's case history and physical condition before
a skin disease is called intrinsic.

The detection

To find out the cause or causes of allergic eczema,
the physician plans a series of patch tests, but only
after a careful study of the patient's history. The
series includes any suspected allergens in the
patient's home or his place of work, any food which
he often eats, and any drugs which he takes
regularly.

After the tests have been made, the allergist reads
the results. He adds these readings to what he
already knows from the case history and the
physical examination. In all probability, one of the
three will have pointed out certain things that must
be eliminated by the patient. These are then
removed, either from the diet or from contact.

For a rare case

Suppose you are one of those rare cases in which
the allergen still has not been discovered. Your
physician then begins a trial-and-error method.

If he suspects that a pollen is the guilty allergen,
he may tell you to change your surroundings and
seek a new environment. This can be very revealing
in searching for the guilty substance. He may also
give you skillfully planned diets which enable him to
eliminate entire groups of foods from your daily
menu with absolutely no injury to your health or
discomfort in your natural eating habits. If a

particular diet makes your eczema appear, he begins to eliminate foods in the group from your menu one at a time. He studies the effects of removing each of the foods until he can put his finger on the exact cause of your eczema.

For immediate relief

Your physician will prescribe suitable lotions or ointments to reduce the discomfort of eczema. Nevertheless, any lasting comfort only comes from finding the exact cause.

Contact dermatitis

As the term suggests, this disease concerns only those allergens which can touch the skin. When you consider the enormous variety of objects touched, handled, worn, and used every day, you get an idea of how many possible allergens there are in existence.

The first symptoms are redness with extreme itching. Shortly, these are followed by swelling, blisters, weeping, and crust formation. Pus appears in the blisters if infection becomes an added factor. But, contact dermatitis may resemble many other skin conditions from which it must be differentiated.

Everyday things such as leather, fabrics, furs, and drugs may be the allergens, whether they are present in the home or are used in an occupation.

Among certain allergic people skin disorders result from all kinds and colors of leather articles. Shoes, jackets, purses, gloves, golf clubs, key-holders, hats, watchbands, and wallets cause skin diseases or allergies. In most of these cases, the allergen is an agent used in tanning, finishing, dyeing, or, more recently, in preventing mildew. The finishes contain resins, fish, and castor oil. In the dyes, all colors may be suspected, particularly brown and black. Anti-mildew substances often contain derivatives of carbolic acid. Chemicals and dyes used in the manufacture of leather reach the skin when they are dissolved by perspiration or when the article becomes soaked with water while on the body.

In addition to real leather, the expanding use of artificial leather has increased the number of persons allergic to the ingredients of which these synthetics are composed. Therefore, such products as vegetable oils, cotton fabrics, rubber, paper, felt, and sulfur become possible contact allergens.

When there's a rash on your feet, look at your shoes!

Whether shoes are made of artificial or genuine leather, the backs or the linings may also be responsible for wheals, redness, and itching.

Remember that patch tests in shoe dermatitis are more helpful when pieces of leather from the tongue of the shoe and from the inner linings are used.

In some people, the rash closely resembles ringworm.

Contact dermatitis from clothing

As in shoe dermatitis, the allergens that cause sensitivity to clothing are substances used in dyeing and processing the cloth. There have been a few cases of symptoms from touching raw silk and wool, but these are fairly rare.

Although numerous articles of clothing cause

allergic dermatitis, sensitivity to dresses is most frequent. Through contact, many colors and all kinds of fabrics may produce symptoms. Dresses made of silk, wool, cotton, nylon, and even glass may produce allergic reactions. The guilty colors in the spectrum of allergy range from white to black.

Three factors involved in "dress dermatitis" are obesity, the amount of perspiration, and the type of perspiration. While persons of all ages are affected by this disease, there are more cases among middle-aged women. Often, these sensitized persons use a great number of deodorants, depilatories, and shaving materials. Use of these products undoubtedly complicates the trouble.

Symptoms first appear where the clothing touches the skin. The armpits may react severely. Harriet D. had a case of dress dermatitis. Miss D. first noticed symptoms of a skin disease around her armpits, neck, chest, abdomen, back, and thighs. She found no signs of allergy on the skin of her legs, feet, and hands. The affected areas were red and itching. Crusty and running sores developed, too. Harriet's symptoms are those of myriads of women who suffer from the same kind of allergy.

When questioned, the patient often suspects or identifies the guilty article of clothing. Here again, you see the value of a complete case history. A patch test with the material in question will either prove or disprove the patient's suspicion. Allergists have come across extreme cases where a patient reacts to as many as thirteen different shades and colors and to six to eight dress materials. Many substances, such as those used in synthetic processing of materials, may be added to the long list of dyes that cause allergic dermatitis.

Although, in most cases, symptoms appear

shortly after the dress is worn for the first time, they will usually disappear completely if the garment isn't used again within a few weeks. Like all allergies, the more often the victim is exposed to the allergen, the longer the symptoms last, and the worse they become.

Certain people are only allergic to an article of clothing the first time they wear it. Some materials lose all of their excess dye after they are washed and no longer cause symptoms. Washable shirts, pajamas, and dresses belong in this group. Some allergic patients stay free of skin disorders as long as they remember to launder all their new washable garments before wearing them.

The best way to avoid a skin allergy to a fabric is by testing a piece of the material in question before wearing it. If this precaution is impossible, reactions can be avoided by buying only those fabrics, colors, and shades which you have worn before without discomfort.

In addition to fabric dermatitis from dresses, an allergic person may react to scarfs, stockings, girdles, gloves, underwear, and coats. Where an allergy to coats is present, waterproofing, crease-holding, and anti-mildew chemicals may be the allergens.

Furs, furbelows, feathers, and furniture

Closely associated with coat dermatitis is allergy to furs. It is the dye in the fur, rather than the pelt itself, which causes skin dermatitis. With the production of low-priced fur coats in recent years, the problem has increased. Attractive commercial names are given to skins so that many people who are allergic to rabbit buy coats made of rabbit without being aware of it. Knowing your fur can be just as great an asset in fighting allergy as it is in getting a bargain.

Although not a fabric or a fur, jewelry is classified with clothing, and causes skin diseases among people who are allergic to nickel, cobalt, platinum, chromium, and gold. These metals are used in rings, watches, bracelets, earrings, spectacle frames, and in an enormous number of trimmings. Rashes caused by metals appear on the neck, arms, fingers, face, or wherever the jewelry is worn.

Occasionally, a case of allergy to feather trimmings is found. The frequency of these cases depends on the current fashion trend in women's clothing. During seasons in which feather-trimmed evening gowns, negligees, hats, and bed jackets are popular, the number of skin reactions to feathers naturally increases.

More often, though, the feathers which cause symptoms are found in cushions, pillows, mattresses, and other types of bedding.

The patient can usually identify the article to which he is allergic by associating the time when his symptoms began with the clothing or bedding he used or touched.

A reaction to furniture may be caused by a sensitivity to feathers or to a fabric. Other materials are paint, lacquer, varnish, and metal trimmings.

Drugs and chemicals

If drugs and chemicals are the allergens, they may be contacted either at work or in the home. Chemists

and drug workers often handle a variety of substances which cause scaling, itching, and inflamed
sores. This type of contact dermatitis is purely
occupational. When a substance is suspected, rubber
gloves should be used to protect the hands from
further contact.

But large numbers of ointments and salves used in
the home may contain drugs and chemicals which
cause allergies, also. Since most people who buy
patent medicines have no idea of their ingredients
and the hazards involved in usage, they should be
extremely careful in the application of these products.

"Cosmetic dermatitis"

Many people have an allergy to cosmetics—a type
of contact dermatitis. This is found most often
among beauty operators who handle hair dyes, hair
wavers, hair straighteners, soaps, tars, and petro-
leum oils. This is to be expected since they constantly
handle an enormous variety of beauty preparations
in the course of their work.

Less frequently, the workers who are employed in
the manufacture of cosmetics suffer from this
disease. The largest number of allergic patients,
however, are everyday users of these products.

All cosmetics are tested in the laboratory before
they are distributed for sale. However, the newest
beauty preparations may produce skin reactions
more often than the older ones, because they may
contain substances to which the user has not been
previously exposed. Therefore, before any manufacturer places a new face powder, lipstick, or other

beauty aid on the market, he should do four things:

(1) Examine the product in the laboratory to find out if it contains any ingredients which would irritate a healthy skin.

(2) Make patch tests and study the results.

(3) Watch the results when the product is used in everyday life.

(4) Change the formula if found harmful.

Several hundred persons should be given patch tests with the new product. These tests are read at the end of 48 hours, and each day for three days thereafter. Two weeks after the last reading, the whole process should be repeated. If any rash or redness appears in more than one percent of those tested, the product should not be distributed.

In addition, an old, reliable, and established beauty aid should be selected and compared to the new product, by subjecting it to all the same tests as the new one.

Ingredients in toiletries and cosmetics that may cause allergy

Various chemicals such as sulfides and alkalies are necessary in manufacturing depilatories but they may cause skin irritation. Alkalies and certain chemicals derived from carbolic acid are the allergens in soap and cleansers. Hair preparations contain dyes, carbolic acid, and perfumes which cause skin rashes in some individuals. Other ingredients used in cosmetics which may either enhance your beauty or give you skin rashes are copper, orris root, mercury, resins, and genuine or artificial oils of flowers. The indelible dyes are more likely to affect one's skin than non-indelible dyes. Some cases do result, though, from the various lake (water soluble) colors.

Symptoms and course of cosmetic dermatitis

The symptoms vary as much as the offending allergens. Swelling is common, although not always present. The affected part is red and irritated. In some people, wheals (like mosquito bites) are the only symptom. In others, the skin which contacts the cosmetic or toiletry becomes dry and scaly. Unless such skin is treated, it will crack, peel, and may discharge pus. In the majority of cases, there is extreme itching. This is, perhaps, the most nerve-wracking symptom of skin allergy.

Cosmetic dermatitis usually begins on that part of the body where the preparation is used. Allergy to rouge, face powder, or face creams is limited to the face and neck. Reactions to deodorants first appear under the arms. After a prolonged period, the skin irritation and wheals show a tendency to spread over larger areas of the body.

All of these symptoms become more uncomfortable in warm, humid weather. If the patient is obese, careless about bathing, or perspires excessively, the reactions are more severe. Nervousness and an unhealthy mental outlook may also increase the discomforts of allergy.

Your general physical condition must be considered, too. Lack of sleep, poor food, and overindulgence in alcohol, tobacco, or food all combine to make a person more susceptible to any allergen.

Detecting the allergen

First, a number of patch tests may be performed. The tests include all of those cosmetics which the allergy patient uses regularly.

The second and preferable method is for the patient to use the suspected cosmetic or toiletry for four or five days, applying it as usual. In this way, the allergist follows the effects of the preparation on the skin.

Many manufacturers refuse to make public the contents of their beauty preparations. If such a preparation proves to be an allergen, a competent chemical analysis may be necessary to find out which of the product's ingredients causes the sensitivity. The patient may find another brand that does not contain the allergen and so may continue to use cosmetics. A change of products prevents sensitivity in most cases. And many products are made especially for those prone to cosmetic dermatitis.

Contact dermatitis from use of household detergents

Any householder takes a sensible precaution in wearing rubber gloves while washing dishes or clothes by hand. Polishes, dry cleaners, and almost anything you use around the house may cause contact dermatitis. Protect your hands!

The type of medicine depends on the symptoms

There are many ointments, powders, oils, and other preparations for direct use on the skin to help soothe and relieve the irritated condition. But the kind of medicine to be used depends on the type of symptoms. If Mrs. A.'s skin is red, itching, and burning, an ordinary bath powder, or one containing boric acid, will help.

Miss B. has patches of crusty sores. Her condition is improved by using an ointment containing menthol, camphor, or coal tar.

Mr. C.'s moist, running sores are a constant source of discomfort. A solution of boric acid will relieve his discomfort.

In severe cases, steroid preparations may do wonders.

Poison ivy and other plants that cause contact dermatitis

Few people, with the possible exception of those who live in the ice-covered areas of the Far North and the Far South, have not been exposed to poison ivy. An estimated 75 percent of the adults in the United States are allergic to this plant. In fact, so many millions of people have reacted to poison ivy that many doubt that this skin disorder is an allergic one. But research has demonstrated that new-born infants and Eskimos, both of whom had never been previously exposed, did not react to poison ivy. A person must be exposed to ivy at least once before he reacts to it. After the first exposure, he will react on further contact with the plant.

Touching the plant is only one of the many ways in which exposure occurs. Some people show severe symptoms when they are near the smoke of burning ivy. Serious cases have even resulted when articles of clothing, such as shoes, boots, gloves, and coats, touched the skin months after that time when the ivy was smeared on these articles. Dogs, cats, and horses who have brushed against the plant may give the disease to persons who later come in contact with them.

Also, several hundred plants other than poison ivy can cause skin diseases. Therefore, all plants which cause skin allergies are considered in diagnosing plant dermatitis. The major plant allergens, in addition to poison ivy, are poison oak, poison sumac, Japanese lacquer, liquid from the shell of the cashew nut, Indian marking nut, and the bulbs of the tulip, gladiolus, geranium, and chrysanthemum.

Poison ivy symptoms and course

If you are exposed to one of these plants, your symptoms usually run the following course:

The disease begins with a rash, redness, itching, and blisters at the site where your skin touched the plant. The blisters break easily and run. Because the liquid in the blisters contains the allergen, the blisters spread quickly along the face, arms, and legs. You must take great care not to scratch or the disease will spread rapidly.

These symptoms usually show up after you have been on a hike, picnic, or fishing trip in an area where the plant grows. The blisters and itching occur from about 24 to 48 hours after exposure to the plant. At first, discomfort is felt only at the site of contact.

Whether or not the disease spreads depends upon how severe your attack is, how quickly you have it treated, and to what extent you cooperate with your physician.

The rash reaches its peak within five to seven days. It gradually disappears after a week or ten days. The time will vary, of course, with the severity of the disease and the kind of care you receive.

Not all cases of plant dermatitis can be traced to a single outing or to a single exposure. Floyd V. is an example. His symptoms are chronic; they last for months. Since none of the common plants are in bloom when his symptoms appear, the seasonal allergens must be dismissed. From a careful examination of Mr. V., the allergist knows Floyd's contact with the allergen is frequent. His discomfort is continuous. Therefore Floyd's skin reactions are caused by a plant which he handles often. Floyd is a florist and his is an occupational allergy to tulip bulbs which he handles in his shop.

But despite the various ways in which contact may be made, the skin reactions are about the same. We still find the itching, rash, and blisters. In Mr. V.'s case, treatment of the skin rash and the use of rubber gloves when handling tulip bulbs prevented recurrences.

Diagnosing plant dermatitis

If plant dermatitis appears after an outing in the country or, as is frequent among children, on arrival at summer camp, the allergen can usually be identified quickly by testing the common allergens. Continuous symptoms require testing of the plants in the individual's home and those he handles at work. This method is the most reliable method of tracing and identifying the guilty allergen. The patch test is used to do this.

Applications for comfort

Treatment of plant dermatitis does not only consist of removing the allergen from contact. There are a number of "on-the-spot" skin applications that make the patient more comfortable. Effective relief from the rashes caused by poison ivy and other plants is obtained by applying boric acid solutions (with or without camphor water) or Burow's powder dissolved in water. The latter drug is particularly beneficial when the blisters continually run.

The soothing, cooling effect these dressings have are due to the evaporation of the liquid. Because of this, a thick, porous cloth that will not dry too quickly is used for these applications. The cloth is soaked with the solution and placed directly against the diseased skin. The treatment is continued until the skin heals sufficiently and stops itching.

Injections of ivy extract or other plant extracts are of no value; they may even aggravate the condition. Injectible steroids may be used, however.

Along with the local treatment, one bath per day is permissible. The water should be near body temperature and only a small amount of castile soap may be used. No vigorous scrubbing is permitted. The body should be dried by patting with a soft towel. Excessive rubbing with a bath towel will prolong and spread the attack and increase the itching.

Preparation is much better than disease

If you are allergic to a seasonal plant, your allergist will help you be prepared for the seasonal attack. He tries to immunize you, by injection, to your allergen.

The injection methods vary in their effectiveness with each person. The immunity they provide is usually temporary and they should be repeated every year, unless—or until—the symptoms disappear. They are extremely helpful among people who for reasons of family responsibility or work cannot move away from an area where their plant allergen grows.

There are still other ways to help prevent plant dermatitis. Certain protective ointments can be applied before any possible exposure. Florists and others who must handle plants can wear rubber gloves.

Help yourself!

Whether the allergens which affect the skin are cosmetic, eczematous, plant, or any of the other types, a necessary ingredient of all cures is general care, which includes the many, many things every patient can do to help himself.

One factor that affects any skin disease is diet. If you have a sensitivity, be sure your diet is free from allergic foods. Include vitamins, minerals, fresh fruits and vegetables, meat, and milk in planning your meals. Do not eliminate a food unless you are sure that it is harmful. The removal of a valuable food from your diet is dangerous because it deprives an already overtaxed system of the vital elements needed to fight disease. Prolonged self-prescribed diets are just as capable of injuring the body as a skin disease.

Of course, in your zest for well-planned meals, you must not eat a food to which you know you are allergic or one which your physician has prohibited. Instead, substitute a food which has the same value as the restricted one. Substances which increase the flow of blood to the skin must be avoided. Fortunately, the foods and drinks in this group, if eliminated, will not cause any dietary deficiency. They include curry, black pepper, mustard, horseradish, and other condiments. Among the liquids are tea, coffee, and alcoholic beverages.

If you are underweight or obese, you should pay special attention to the problem of bringing your weight to normal.

Closely associated with diet is the problem of constipation. The best method of relieving constipation is always through the use of foods rather than drugs. Roughage, such as a daily intake of bran, plenty of water, and fruit juices will probably suffice.

As has already been discussed, bathing is both permissible and desirable if you suffer from an allergic skin disease. Don't scrub or rub the skin vigorously. Only very small amounts of mild soap should be used, and often plain water is more advisable. All bath water must be as near to body temperature as possible to prevent an increase in itching.

Any of these rules for general care, once prescribed, can be followed with little difficulty. All patients will be pleasantly surprised by the extent to which they can help themselves.

Chapter VIII
GUIDELINES FOR PARENTS

Although there are special problems in treating allergies of infants and children, the picture is by no means bleak. Nearly all children respond well to allergic treatment. The saddest cases are those infants and children who have *not* been treated, the children who have become chronic invalids unnecessarily.

Parents who understand the allergic child's problems and how to cope with them are not only going to benefit the child, but will lead more tranquil lives themselves.

A word about prevention

First of all, because allergy tends to run in families—even though specific diseases are not inherited—children of allergic parents should not be exposed unnecessarily to sensitizing agents—dogs, cats, stuffed toys, and inhalants. These children should be observed for early signs of allergy. If any signs appear, treatment should begin immediately.

A child is a child

More important than the fact that your child is an allergic child is the fact that he is a child. The child who needs specialized care also needs the normal attentions of a nonallergic child. Because he is a special case, he may need them more.

The allergic child needs parental approval, the assurance that his parents are kind to him because he is their child—not because he is allergic.

Is an allergic child a neurotic child?

Of course some neurotic children are also allergic. But there is no definite evidence favoring the idea that childhood allergy is more frequently psychosomatic than other diseases.

Yet, the child who goes to school with eczema on his face, the child with perennial rhinitis, who is constantly sniffling and blowing, the child who can never play long with others because of his asthma, has special problems in dealing with his playmates. He may be shunned, or made fun of.

Such a child may become overly self-conscious, haunted by constant fears of his affliction. He may develop a feeling of inferiority or become intensely disagreeable. The asthmatic may form the habit of apologizing in advance for asthma attacks that never occur.

Another allergic child can have parents who are so

anxious to do everything possible for him that they are overattentive and never say "no." As he grows up, his appetite for attention increases, and his tolerance of anyone who says "no" to him decreases.

It is clear that allergy can easily lay the groundwork for neurosis, and that this is more likely than the other way around.

Again, one of the best ways to avoid these problems is to get early treatment for the allergic child.

Is an allergic child a behavior problem?

The logical answer to this question, and to others like it, is, "Let's take one child at a time." In other words, extreme general conclusions can lead to irreparable harm. The safest way, and the way that works, is to examine the special problems of each child and deal cooperatively with all persons who can help him. False divisions into "emotional," "physical," and "behavioral," can lead only to further confusion.

Can he outgrow his allergy?

No.

Suppose your child has eczema. Do you think that by the time he is fourteen or fifteen the eczema will have disappeared? You may be entirely wrong. In fact, the eczema may have spread and become more unsightly. We have already talked about the social distress and harm that may come from this condition.

Suppose you are the parent of an asthmatic child.

If you do little about it, and hope for the best, will your child wake up one morning without asthma? Hardly. More likely, he may become a chronic invalid.

Can he be cured?

Although allergy cannot be completely obliterated, it can certainly be diminished to the point where it is "almost" cured.

Undoubtedly, this is frustrating to the allergic child and his parents. It is discouraging to face endless years of treatment and regimen. Bear in mind, however, that the allergy itself, if left untreated, is far more unpleasant than the treatment. In a child, especially, it can leave both physical and emotional scars.

Visiting the physician

The chances are that the allergic child will be spending many hours in the physician's office.

Thus, it is important that both parent and child adjust to their visits with the doctor. There is no reason why these visits cannot be relaxed and constructive.

The first visit is always significant, since it may set the pattern for all subsequent visits. The parent should make careful preparations for the first visit. He or she should consult with the doctor or his nurse to decide the best time to bring the child to the office.

The appointment time will hinge on many factors: the child's eating patterns, his nap time, the type of allergy, the doctor's availability, etc. Working together, doctor and parent can arrange a time that is most satisfactory and least disruptive to the child. Haphazard arrangements are likely to backfire and produce negative results.

Many physicians work with children on a regular basis. They know the various methods of establishing a positive relationship with the child, as well as what pitfalls to avoid. The allergic child will probably never look forward with glee to his visits to the office; no child does. But there is no reason why these visits cannot be pleasant and emotionally painless.

Physician and parent

The relationship of the doctor and the parent is as important as that between doctor and child. In certain respects, it is even more important.

The parent must tell the doctor about the child's eating habits, his sleeping habits, the type of clothing he wears, and similar details. In addition, he or she must discuss matters of a personal nature, such as information about the pregnancy, his or her feelings toward the child, toward the spouse, etc.

Will this be an embarrassment? No. When you talk to your physician you are talking to a man who has listened to countless problems, some of them very much like your own. He is trained to handle them in a most sensitive manner, and where they relate to his specialty, to give counsel.

Usually, the physician will allow the parent time to discuss the allergic child in a free and unfettered manner. This will give the parent a chance to disclose the things which are troubling him or her the most. It will also give the doctor a good idea of what questions will be most important.

After the parent's initial explanation, the physician will begin his specific, thorough questioning. In this phase of history-taking, he will try to pin down exact dates. He may request the time of day when attacks occur, what the child was doing, and many other relevant details. Only by persistent questioning can the doctor determine what kind of examination is needed for the child. The parent's full cooperation with the doctor facilitates treatment for the child.

The doctor is likely to try to establish hereditary factors—who in the family has had allergies. He may ask many questions about the pregnancy and whether the child was breast-fed.

He will ask about the child's environment, whether he has brothers and sisters, and what his father's occupation is (or his mother's). Other questions will deal, of course, with the symptoms of the child.

The parent will be encouraged to take notes during this initial interview. There may be questions which he or she may want to ask on the next visit and these notes will serve as handy reminders. This question-and-answer process between parent and doctor is a vital part of most visits.

Another important point. The parent should bring along a friend whom the child trusts and who can take care of the child while parent and doctor discuss the essential problems during this first visit.

After the interview, the doctor is ready to examine the child.

The examination

Sometimes the first visit can last as long as an hour and a half. Although there are numerous exceptions to this rule, it is better to enter the office prepared for a long stay than to fidget and fuss because of a conflicting engagement.

If the doctor feels that the illness is indeed caused by an allergen, his task is just beginning. Using every technique at his command, he must search out the offending allergen from a host of pretenders.

Progress notes

The discussions between doctor and parent are not finished after the first visit.

In order for these discussions to be as helpful as possible to the child, doctors have devised a method of obtaining accurate information from parents regarding the child's progress. This method is called "progress notes."

This means that the parent has to pay close attention to the reactions of the child to skin tests, medications, foods, etc. At the start of each visit, or when necessary, he or she informs the doctor of all pertinent facts. Physicians often keep a "progress chart" of the child to facilitate this phase of the treatment.

An important result of progress notes is the education of the parent. As the parent continues to increase his or her knowledge of the subject, he or she becomes a valuable ally in the fight against allergic disease.

Chapter IX

INFANTS' ALLERGIES

Food allergens and substitutes

Among allergic infants, egg and milk products are the foods that most often cause allergic symptoms. This is not surprising, since they are the foods which comprise most of the baby's diet from the time he is born.

When milk or one of its by-products bring on an allergy, either whey or casein (the curd) is the allergen. Whey is the liquid part of the curdled milk. Although you cannot see it in fresh milk, it is there. Casein is a protein in the curd of the milk. Occasionally, a child is sensitive to both casein and whey.

The infant may be fed on human, goat's, or mare's milk instead of cow's milk if whey alone is the allergen. Canned, evaporated milk from the cow is also used, provided it has been boiled five to ten minutes before the baby drinks it. Also, the allergen can be taken out of fresh cow's milk by boiling it for six hours. Boiling, however, destroys vitamin C. This vitamin must be added to the baby's diet to prevent him from developing a vitamin C deficiency.

There are a number of soybean milks available if natural milks cannot be used. They can be substituted in the baby's bottle after having been cooked for forty-five minutes. There is a possibility that the infant may be allergic to soybean milk as well as to natural milk. For this reason, the baby must be carefully watched if his formula is made with soybean milk.

On the whole, the whey-sensitive patients are much less difficult to treat than those who are allergic to casein. The latter must avoid all milk, whether it is in liquid form or contained in any food. In such cases, the infant is fed a thin porridge to which vitamins, minerals, fats, and proteins have been added. Again, as in whey-sensitive babies, the soybean milks may be used. Other milk substitutes which may be used are the various amino-acid preparations. These products are most helpful in the very young patients who, as yet, are unaware of the rather unpleasant taste and odor of many amino-acid substances. Research has shown that this milk substitute can be used to feed the baby for a long period of time with no harmful effects upon his weight or his nutrition.

Care must be taken, after a change in milk has been made, not to feed the baby any soups, custards, ice creams, or candies containing dried or whole milk of the cow.

Eggs

A much easier allergy to treat than that of sensitivity to milk is sensitivity to eggs. Both raw and cooked egg must be avoided in the baby's diet. This is a fairly easy task. A more difficult problem is to eliminate egg from the diet of a nursing mother. Because the allergen can be carried to the breast-fed baby through the mother's milk, the nursing mother must eliminate all foods such as waffles, pancakes, French toast, muffins, macaroons, cakes, meringues, puddings, sauces, icings, pastas, mayonnaise, and ice creams, if they contain eggs. Sometimes the person who is allergic to eggs may show symptoms when he eats cooked, fried, baked, or boiled chicken.

Other indirect sources of the egg allergen are the vaccines which prevent typhoid, influenza, and yellow fever. Chick embryos are used in making these vaccines. To prepare them a tiny bit of shell is taken from an incubated egg. Typhoid or yellow fever germs are placed inside the egg. Then the shell is replaced and the egg is sealed so that the germs can multiply. Later, the egg is opened and the contents used to manufacture vaccines. Thus, when the baby is vaccinated, he may show the same symptoms as he would from eating an egg.

Fish products

Other food allergies are those to fish products. For example, a baby who reacts to fish may show symptoms by merely inhaling the odor of fish being cooked, even though he eats none of it. Also, he may come in contact with his allergen by licking fish glue off his toys.

Bacteria

The other common allergen among infants is bacteria. Any mild infection of the tonsils, sinuses, ears, nose, lungs, or bronchial tubes exposes the patient to bacteria. After a time, the baby becomes sensitive to the bacteria. Allergic symptoms appear and soon the child not only has a bodily infection but a serious allergy.

Contactants and inhalants

Sometimes babies are allergic to materials they touch or inhale. Mattress and pillow stuffings of felt and feathers may cause allergic reactions. Bed clothing and dust may be other offenders.

The common allergic diseases of infancy: asthma

Asthma can begin as early as the first weeks of life. In eight out of ten asthma cases, especially in infants and in children, there is a family history of allergy of some kind.

A mild infection in a baby's ear or throat may send him into the throes of asthma with the same wheezing and gasping present in adult cases. These symptoms come within a few days after the first infection. They appear so quickly and are so severe that they are often frightening. Once the infection is treated, relief comes quickly.

Bacteria and inhalants are the major causes. But,

asthma often appears simultaneously with an unexplained skin or food allergy, and frequently comes in the winter. During the weeks or months between attacks the baby is apt to be completely free of symptoms. The asthma may disappear during the first four or five years of his life and return again when the child reaches the age of eleven or twelve.

Eczema (atopic dermatitis)

The surface of the baby's skin is affected. This, in general, itches, burns, scales, weeps, and reddens. But the number and type of skin symptoms vary with the individual. One baby will have only a mild rash with slight itching and redness while another will suffer from a group of large, yellow, waxy sores that exude a watery fluid. It usually begins on the face, scalp, and neck, but it may spread over the entire body if it is neglected. Infections, foods, and materials touched may all be causative.

If you are a parent and suspect that your child has the wet type of eczema, look for the following signs: crusting, running sores on the scalp, neck, and face, particularly the cheeks. The nose and chin are usually free of the disease even though the rest of the face is affected. Some babies have the symptoms on the small of the back and around the sex organs. Wherever the disease appears, the itching is intense. Very often, except for the eczema, the patient's general condition is good.

If the physician suspects the dry group of eczema, he looks for fine scabs on the skin surrounded by bright red patches. Swelling may or may not accompany this condition.

Allergic reactions within the baby's system

These do not appear as frequently as asthma or eczema, but, when they do occur, they are extremely painful. When the allergen, generally a food, is swallowed, the baby's tongue, lips, and face swell. He has nausea and vomits. In addition, a skin rash, asthma, abdominal pain, and diarrhea are other symptoms. In many cases, the offending food is or contains eggs, milk, or fish products. Obviously, every possible precaution should be taken in having the baby avoid these allergens.

Treating the allergic baby

This is not as difficult as for older children and adults. The baby has a regulated diet and controlled surroundings. A complete discussion of these with the allergist helps him to find the cause of the trouble and to prevent further exposure.

Avoiding the allergen, whenever possible, is the best method of treating a food allergy. There are many nonallergenic products now on the market to replace bedding, pillows, or other materials that may be causing trouble.

General health measures should be taken, too. This means not taking the baby to motion-picture houses and stores which are often overheated and poorly ventilated as well as attended by people suffering from a variety of diseases. Subways, buses, trains, and all other modes of public transportation are a threat to the health of the very young, also. Although fresh air and sunshine are vital to the physical being of the infant, the places where he is taken should be carefully selected to protect him from unnecessary exposure.

Chapter X
CHILDHOOD ALLERGIES

Unlike the allergies of infancy, the allergies of childhood include almost all of those suffered by adults. But, the most common allergy among children is asthma. It accounts for about half of all chronic illness in childhood. The U.S. Public Health Service has estimated that more than two million children sixteen years of age and younger have asthma, either steadily or in episodes from time to time. A quarter of the school absenteeism and of the restricted activity of school-age children can be attributed to asthma.

Hay fever may be the first sign of allergy in childhood. Because the attacks are mild, parents may dismiss them as a "summer cold" or as an ailment which will be outgrown. However, a large percentage of mild hay fever symptoms are often mere preludes to asthma. Thus, the sneezing, running, and itching and redness of the nose and eyes that are caused by hay fever may develop into shortness of breath, wheezing, and other symptoms of asthma.

Whether a child's hay fever develops suddenly or gradually into severe asthma, there are usually two explanations: (1) The organs in the body that react to allergy have changed. In other words, the bronchial tubes have also acquired the sensitivity which was formerly in the eyes. (2) An infection has begun.

Among children's allergies, sensitivity to pollens, house dust, animal hair and saliva, and foods are most frequent.

Asthma

Asthma in children is the same disease as that in adults. Fortunately, most can have it controlled. For those in school, medication taken just before participating in active exercise often prevents attacks.

The most serious type of attack, status asthmaticus, a static attack, or one that lasts a particularly long time, leads to deprivation of oxygen and requires emergency treatment. This does not occur often in children, but is more apt to occur in those who have not received proper care and treatment.

The symptoms of asthma from bacteria are usually not as severe in the child as in the infant, but they last longer. There may be a slight fever, difficult breathing, and wheezing. The attacks may last several days or a week. They may come and go.

After the allergen is discovered, the preferred method of treatment is merely to avoid the allergen, especially in children under six years of age. In older children, desensitizing can be highly effective. The allergist fits injections of extracts of the allergens to the patient's sensitivity and tolerance.

Asthmatic bronchitis

Like asthma, asthmatic bronchitis affects the bronchial tubes. The main symptom is a steady, persistent cough deep in the chest. Wheezing may also be present, as well as labored breathing, but generally these symptoms do not develop until the child has been coughing quite a bit.

The cough is dry in the initial stages, but gets phlegmy as the condition runs its course. Sometimes the phlegm is swallowed, and this leads to nausea and vomiting. Because vomiting activates the mucus in the bronchial tubes, this can have beneficial results. Asthmatic bronchitis can lead to an asthmatic condition. The disease may be seasonal or occur throughout the year.

Chronic allergic cough

This allergic irritation develops in the upper respiratory tract. The symptoms are easy to recognize: coughing and more coughing. Unlike asthmatic bronchitis, the cough remains dry. This condition also may be seasonal or occur throughout the year.

Skin diseases

Infections are the cause of much skin disease in children, as well as of asthma. Often an infected sinus, a boil, or some other infection may make the child allergic to bacteria or some other infectious agent. An infection may precede a skin eruption by a few days or weeks.

In other cases, the skin disease either follows or accompanies asthma, hay fever, or other allergic manifestations. A weakened part of the body is more susceptible to allergy than a healthy one.

Other allergens causing skin disease are food, drugs, and contactants. Children are subject to urticaria (hives) and contact dermatitis just as adults are.

In tracking down an offending allergen, children's likes and dislikes of food should be taken into consideration. As mentioned previously, a child often avoids a food to which he is allergic.

Eczema

Eczema or atopic dermatitis in children may be a recurrence from that in the infantile state, or it may develop independently. The rash is usually dry, scaly, thickened, pigmented, and, often, wrinkled. Usually involved are the face, forehead, eyelids, ears, neck, chest, the bends of the forearms, and the backs of the knees and wrists. The itching is extremely intense. Because of scratching and irritation, the skin thickens and a secondary infection may result with scabs and a yellowish discharge.

Physical allergy

After a child has been mildly exposed to the rays of the sun, large crusty blisters may appear on the skin. This is not sunburn. They may appear a few seconds after exposure. The sores occur on both hands, both legs, or both sides of the face, and they weep. "Summer rashes" may also be caused by the heat from a radiator, a hot water bottle, or an electric pad.

If the skin is allergic to cold, an ice pack, snow, or just plain cold weather affect it in the same way. Light, heat, or cold sensitivity show the same symptoms in the child who reacts to any of the three.

Physical allergy is the term applied to allergies caused by heat, cold, or the sun.

Serum sickness

Serum sickness is one of the most dangerous skin allergies of childhood. It may follow injections for tetanus, typhoid, yellow fever, scarlet fever, or any other inoculation to prevent disease. The rash may be red in color or pale and yellowish. The patches vary from the size of a pin to the size of the palm.

The first signs of the rash appear at the site of the injection. The rash may then spread over the entire body. One type lasts from one to three days. The rash is widespread.

Another type is extremely hard to tell from scarlet fever because of the fever and rash. In still another type of serum sickness, the joints become so sore and cause so much pain that the disease resembles lockjaw. In these cases, the jaw, neck, and back become sore and stiff. Another skin reaction looks exactly like measles but, unlike measles, there is no inflammation of the linings of the nose.

In one child, a combination of rashes that looks like scarlet fever in one part of the body, measles in another place, and lockjaw symptoms in still a third area may be found.

Itching and fever are common in all types of serum sickness. The temperature ranges from near normal to 104°. The skin eruptions last from several hours to two weeks. The length of time that symptoms remain depends on the quantity of serum injected in the first dose. Most rashes are bright red, rose, or violet. In overtired patients, or in prolonged cases, the sores are pale and yellowish.

If you are the mother of a child who has once

suffered this disease, don't allow your child to be vaccinated in the future without consulting your physician.

Poison ivy

This is a frequent cause of skin allergy among children. They are exposed to it in parks, at summer camps, on hikes, and in many other ways. As was discussed previously, touching any part of the plant or inhaling the smoke where it is being burned is enough to cause running, itching, and stinging blisters. The discharge from these sores carries the allergen with it and further affects the skin it touches.

To prevent the disease, the child should be taught to recognize the plant and avoid it. Immediately after an exposure, he should take a bath in strong soap and hot water, followed by an alcohol rub-down. This prevents poison ivy in most cases.

Wet dressings with boric acid can reduce the itching and prevent spread. They cannot cure. The child should be kept from scratching. No treatment can be effective so long as the child continues to scratch. In some cases, the doctor may prescribe a tranquilizer to quiet the child's nerves and make scratching less likely. Antihistamines help control itching, and in severe cases steroid drugs are often extremely helpful.

The type of clothing worn by the child should not be overlooked. The irritation may be caused or aggravated by friction of nylon or woolen clothing against the skin. If you have an eczematous child, try to dress him in soft cotton clothes. Also, if the weather is warm, avoid overdressing. Garments should be loose at all times. Encourage the child to play with his friends. This will make him forget the itching, and also make him physically tired and ready for sleep. In warmer weather, expose the skin to sunlight, always being careful to avoid sunburn.

Chapter XI

MISCELLANEOUS ALLERGIES

Insect stings

When there are more than one hundred thousand species of stinging insects, it is probably surprising that more people are not allergic to bee or other insects' stings. There are as many as twenty thousand species of bees alone. But, serious reactions have been reported to stings of only about thirty of these.

Inhalation of insect scales or dust from the wings and body, injection of the venom through the sting, or instillation of salivary secretion all can cause allergy.

For the unlucky, an insect sting can be especially serious. When symptoms occur throughout the whole body (a systemic reaction), or in places other than the stung area, it is important to find a doctor or go to a hospital at once.

Large hives may appear all over the body. One may experience a feeling of tightness in the throat or chest, dry cough, sneezing, wheezing, rapid pulse, and a fall in blood pressure. Other symptoms are an unusually red or pale skin, a sensation of heat all over the body, and a feeling of uneasiness and fear. Dizziness, nausea, vomiting, cramps, and difficulty in swallowing or breathing follow. All this may happen in a few minutes to a few hours.

This is anaphylactic shock, which may also be caused by a drug or a food to which a person is especially sensitive.

Washing the stung area with soap and water is helpful for any painful sting. To help keep the venom from spreading, ice cubes or ice packs can be applied to the injury. The effected part of the body should be raised to decrease the circulation. An application of meat tenderizer solution to the injury can help destroy the venom.

For those who are sensitive to insect stings

If further contact with stinging insects is likely, you may be desensitized by weekly injections of tiny, measured doses of extracts prepared from doses of pure venom injected into the skin.

If you have had even a mild whole-body reaction to insect sting, wearing a medical identification tag with information on it of your insect sensitivity is an excellent idea.

Naturally, no one, allergic or not, wants to get stung, and these commonsense precautions may easily be taken.

(1) Stay clear of hanging wasp nests and piles of fallen leaves and dead logs that may hide wasp nests. Have any nearby wasp or hornet nests destroyed by a professional exterminator.

(2) Always wear shoes outdoors.

(3) In any insect country, wear close fitting clothes without a rough texture or odor (such as leather). Colors should be subdued.

(4) Remember that scented soap and cosmetics attract insects.

(5) Stay away from flower beds, fields of clover, and orchards full of fresh fruit.

(6) Keep auto windows closed so that insects can't get in.

(7) Spray picnic areas with an insect repellent and keep garbage cans tightly closed. (Food attracts bees and wasps.)

Remember that stinging insects are more likely to attack rapidly moving objects. If, after all these precautions, a bee or wasp buzzes around you or lands on your clothes or skin, stay still, or continue walking slowly. Do not thrash at it.

If you know that you are allergic to insect stings, ask your doctor for a kit to take to picnics or other places where the attention of a doctor or a hospital is not quickly obtainable. (See Part II.)

Headaches

Allergies are the most important factor in many headaches. About 11 percent of migraine cases are due to an allergen. Avoidance of a single food has been known to cure migraine.

Spots before the eyes (scintillating scotoma), or flashes before the eyes are warnings of migraine. A throbbing pain, usually on one side of the head, is often followed by nausea or vomiting. A dull headache and washed-out feeling may last for a day or two afterwards. A combination of aspirin and caffeine at the first warning signs may ward off this type of headache.

When nasal membranes become swollen because of an allergy and block drainage of sinuses, a painful sinus headache can occur. Allergens may also cause an actual swelling of the brain tissue.

Frontal headaches are common locations for allergic headaches and may be accompanied by a stuffy nose. Although foods are the most common offenders, inhalants, such as animal dander, dust, pollen, mold spores, and drugs such as aspirin and phenolphthalein, have all been reported as causes of allergic headache. Among female patients, the attacks may occur at the same time as menstruation.

When an allergy to foods is suspected as a cause of migraine, elimination diets are used to identify the specific allergen. If a drug or inhalant is responsible, skin tests are made. Once the offending substance is discovered, it must be avoided. Many cases of migraine are cured this way.

To treat attacks that appear before or during menstruation, an extract of female hormones is given in gradually increased doses. This treatment has been effective with many women. There is also the possibility of sexual disturbances in males at the time of their attacks.

Menière's Disease

One of the most distressing conditions which

involves the nervous system is "Menière's Disease." The symptoms are deafness, ringing in the ears, dizziness, nausea, vomiting, and jerkiness of the eyeballs. Allergy to milk, wine, plums, vinegar, spinach, pears, wheat, eggs, beef, pork, or any other food may produce Menière's Disease. House dust and orris root can also serve as causes.

Women are approximately eight times as susceptible to the disease as men. Symptoms usually begin at about the age of thirty. The onset is often gradual, appearing as a slight ringing in the ears, difficulty in hearing, irritability, and fatigue. This is followed by severe headaches, dizziness, and finally deafness. Sweating and vomiting may accompany the ear symptoms.

The symptoms just described are typical of all cases of Menière's Disease, although not every individual who suffers from these symptoms is truly allergic. Allergy is but one of the three generally recognized causes. Some cases may be due to a sensitivity to histamine, a substance manufactured by the body when it comes in contact with an allergen. Experiments have shown that a reaction to histamine produces identical symptoms. The treatment consists of gradually increased doses of histamine, two or three times a week, until the maximum amount that can be tolerated is reached. After three months, a second treatment is advisable. You will note the similarity here to the use of allergic extracts to relieve other sensitivities.

Still another cause is the constriction or tightening of the blood vessels, which makes it difficult for the blood to circulate. In such cases, the doctor may inject the patient with nicotinic acid, a vitamin substance, to relax the blood vessels.

Because most cases of Menière's Disease result

from this constriction, a diagnosis of allergy should not be made hastily. The personal and family history of the patient is the first indication of sensitivity. A thorough physical examination either confirms or denies the presence of infections and organic disturbances. Not until these measures are taken is an attempt made to classify the disease as allergic. If the condition appears as a result of a food allergy, skin tests and elimination diets may be necessary. Precautions must be taken to avoid subsequent exposure to any foods which produce symptoms.

Menière's Disease is no minor ailment. Unless it is treated within a reasonable time after the initial attack, permanent deafness may result.

Neuritis

Neuritis is often caused by sensitization of the nerve tissue. Although occasionally cases are the result of allergy to food or to bacteria, most frequently the sensitizers which cause allergic neuritis are serums, particularly tetanus antitoxin.

The regions most often affected are the networks of nerves in the neck, the loins, and the inner side of the hip-bone. The presence of a skin rash is common. There may be either temporary or permanent paralysis. If the affected nerves degenerate, there is little hope for the recovery of the paralyzed areas, but early treatment will avoid this danger.

If the allergen is believed to be a serum, there can be no experimentation because of the extreme danger involved. When drugs or foods are suspected, the use of elimination diets and skin tests often show just what allergen is responsible.

Allergic neuritis can be cured if the treatment is

begun early. The patient is warned against injections of serum and is informed of the harm his food or drug allergens may cause.

Other parts of the body affected by serum sickness are the joints. Indeed, pain in the knees, ankles, elbows, wrists, and the small joints of the hands and feet may be the only symptom felt by a victim of this allergy. The reaction may vary from mild stiffness to a hot, red, swollen, and extremely tender inflammation. The intensity of the disease depends upon how strongly allergic the patient is and how much serum has been injected.

The symptoms are so similar to those of rheumatic fever and arthritis that it is hard to diagnose them as allergic. This is especially true where the joints are involved. A clue to the allergic source of the condition is the presence of pain and stiffness in the joints of the jaw, the sides of the head, and the base of the skull. This stiffness is not as frequent in rheumatic fever as in neuritis, but even this clue may be misleading.

The symptoms in the joints last from a few hours to nine days. They may appear simultaneously with, precede, or follow an allergic skin rash, asthma, or other allergic reactions. Sometimes nausea is present at the same time. As a rule, a person does not experience any discomfort in his joints until two or three days after the onset of the rash.

Allergic eye conditions

A common allergic manifestation, conjunctivitis, may be due to external allergens. Symptoms are extreme itching, burning, tearing, and light-sensitiveness. There may be spasms about the eyes.

The lower lid is usually the more seriously affected with hives, from pinpoint to pinhead in size. Conjunctivitis is often associated with respiratory allergies, hay fever, perennial rhinitis, and asthma. It may occur along with intestinal symptoms if the allergen comes in contact with the eye area. The most severe forms of conjunctivitis are known as vernal catarrh.

Angioedema of the eye structures can occur, and may be due to bedding, feather pillows, woolen coverings, or ice cream.

A condition known as blepharitis is frequently due to a cosmetic. It involves the edge or margin of the eyelids with congestion, scales, and, sometimes, weeping. It is often associated with dandruff of the scalp which may aggravate the condition. To cure the allergy, the scalp must be treated for dandruff.

Bacteria may be responsible for some of these conditions because the individual has become allergic to them. Infections in the teeth, upper respiratory tract—sinuses, tonsils, larynx, and pharynx—or bronchial tubes may be causative.

Whether the eye problem is seasonal or persists indefinitely depends on the causal allergen. If the symptoms are intense, they may outlast the season to which they are normally confined. Daily exposure to an allergen may cause polyps (cauliflower-like growths) to appear on the eye. Eventually, even ulcers may develop.

Not all allergies of the eye are limited to the eyelids. The cornea and iris may be affected as well. The same allergens are responsible for symptoms in these parts of the eyes, with bacteria heading the list.

Hypersensitivity pneumonitis

This is a "newer" allergic disease that has been

known by several different names previously, such as farmer's lung, mushroom worker's disease, and others. The affecting allergens are molds or fungi in contaminated plants, animal products, or other things. It occurs, for instance, among farmers who work with moldy hay and among certain mushroom workers who are in contact with moldy compost.

Symptoms are fever, chills, muscle ache, vague pains in the lower back and knees, shortness of breath, and nonproductive cough. Episodes last from two to five days. Unless the offending allergen is found, exposure to it will make symptoms recur.

Aside from moldy hay and compost, other sources of allergens may be:

> moldy pressed sugarcane (bagasse)
> moldy cork
> contaminated barley
> contaminated maple logs
> contaminated wood dust
> contaminated wood pulp
> contaminated home humidifier and
>   air-conditioning ducts
> pigeon droppings

Home humidifiers should be washed with soap and water weekly and given applications of growth deterrents.

Allergy of the digestive system

This type of allergy may cause nausea, vomiting, diarrhea, salivation, irritation of the stomach, pain in both the stomach and abdomen, gas, and belching. Along with these symptoms, the victim may have swelling of the face, lips, tongue, salivary glands, pharynx, larynx, soft palate, and mucous membranes.

Among infants, recurrent vomiting is common. Though not definitely proved allergic in nature, it frequently occurs among allergic infants. The baby often has fever.

By far the most common digestive allergens are foods: lobster, crab, mackerel, tuna, salmon, beef, pork, chicken, eggs, peas, corn, sweet potatoes, celery, peanuts, Brazil nuts, almonds, honey, and buckwheat. Anything edible is capable of producing allergic symptoms. Aspirin as well as many other drugs may also act as this type of allergen. And again, bacteria may be causative.

In compiling the family and personal history of such a patient, the physician will want to know of any allergy in the parents, the frequency of attacks, the amount of tobacco, drugs, and alcohol consumed, and bowel-movement habits.

The first results of skin tests are not final proof. It is possible for an individual to give a negative reaction to allergens to which he is sensitive, and vice versa, so re-testing is done, if necessary.

A careful physical examination is mandatory in all cases. After the examination, elimination diets may be prescribed if a food is suspected. Foods are withdrawn in groups. Dieting without the help of an allergist is apt to result in serious malnutrition.

Cardiovascular allergies

The allergens that produce symptoms in the heart and blood vessels are food, inhalants, infectious agents such as bacteria, drugs, serum, and physical agents.

Among these, tobacco takes first place. Patients whose hearts "jumped" and "stopped," or beat irregularly, and those who had pains around their hearts, have often found relief by abstaining from smoking. Alcohol has also been proved responsible for similar symptoms.

Infectious agents often cause irregularities in the heart and blood vessels. A person who is allergic to one of them may have asthma, skin rashes, upset stomach, and hay fever as well as an allergic heart condition.

Drugs have caused not only severe allergic attacks, but even fatal ones in a few highly sensitive persons. The same thing is true of serum. Reactions may follow injections of preparations designed to fight tetanus, typhoid, and yellow fever.

Heat and cold

Physical agents, such as heat or cold, may in rare cases be solely responsible for cardiovascular symptoms. The case of Mrs. Ethel D., age 30, is an excellent example of this type of disease. Mrs. D. complained of her "bad heart" and sought medical advice. A thorough physical examination showed that she was in excellent health. An electrocardiograph revealed no organic weakness in her heart. As the examination drew to a close, she made a chance remark that her "heart spells" followed bathing. This casual statement threw an entirely new light on her illness. The possible implications of her chance remark were investigated further and it was found that she was allergic to heat. The hot water in her bath caused the heart irregularities. She began taking baths in lukewarm water and her symptoms disappeared entirely.

Patients have been observed to suffer serious heart attacks when exposed to heat or cold. A hot bath or a cold shower occasionally brings pain and irregularities of the heart. In other cases, this type of allergy, in addition to other allergens, such as food or pollens, produces a highly complicated condition.

Other cardiovascular conditions

Persons with allergies of the heart and blood vessels usually have a lowered skin temperature in the fingers and toes. The blood flow lessens; the pulse and blood pressure increase. These persons are also much more sensitive than average to other allergens and respiratory diseases.

Asthma may accompany cardiovascular symptoms. In some cases, the asthmatic symptoms are the only ones noticed by the patient. If there is a small possibility that the heart is affected during an asthma attack, an electrocardiograph is often advisable. However, it is only during the attack that the electrocardiograph will show any heart irregularity. Before or after the attack, everything usually appears normal.

Treatment

A case history of a person with cardiovascular allergy may reveal tobacco as the allergen. If there is any doubt, however, intradermal tests are made with Maryland burley, Virginia, and Xanthis tobacco. Should these tests be positive, all smoking is prohibited. If the symptoms persist, however, tests must be made for other allergens, such as pollen and other inhalants, or drugs.

When an airborne allergen is found to produce the disease, desensitization of the patient by administration of gradually increased doses of extract is done. Although this method is not practical in extremely severe cases, it often brings relief to victims of mild attacks. The procedure in this treatment is the same as in other forms of allergy. It demands, however, closer observation because of its relation to heart symptoms.

Among food-sensitive individuals who suffer reactions in the heart and blood vessels, a series of elimination diets is the preferred diagnostic tool.

In cases of drug sensitivity, if the reaction is immediate and severe, the identity of the harmful substance is simple. In delayed reactions, tests may be necessary to discover the specific allergen.

If alcohol is the sensitizer, the elimination diet will identify it quickly and it is prohibited at once. Victims of this disease often have phlebitis. Occasionally, an allergy to alcohol is so minor that weak highballs may be taken without ill effects, and only stronger drinks, like cocktails and straight brandy, cause reactions.

Chapter XII
TREATMENT

Treating the allergy involves four factors: the type of allergy, the nature of the allergen, the severity of the allergic reactions, and the complications that accompany the symptoms.

The first step is to compile a case history under the direction of your physician. This includes your symptoms; your environment; any chronic infections you may have; whether attacks are seasonal or perennial; your minor allergic reactions to drugs, foods, or animal danders; how often you are exposed to cosmetics, pets, plants, insecticides, and dusts; the state of your digestion; whether you are constipated or have diarrhea; the presence of headaches and their frequency, duration, and location; your weight; the condition of your teeth; the dates of and reactions to tuberculosis and diphtheria tests and serum injections; and all past and present illnesses, and treatments used.

Along with the case history, a thorough physical examination of the heart, lungs, pelvis, rectum, abdomen, nose, throat, eyes, ears, and teeth is necessary.

Finding the allergen

There are seven tests being used today.

For a highly sensitive patient, the scratch test is often best. This method has the advantage of producing mild reactions only. It is effective in determining allergies to foods, pollens, and animal danders.

The intradermal test is effective in detecting pollen and inhalant allergies.

Patch tests are used to detect chemicals, drugs, clothing, or cosmetics.

In all three of the methods mentioned, the readings are graded as follows: O is negative, + is slight, ++ is moderate, +++ is marked, and ++++ is marked plus. The gradings are determined by the extent of redness and swelling.

When a food is suspected of causing migraine headaches or skin, digestive, heart, or other diseases, elimination diets are used. (See Part II.)

In evaluating the importance of the scratch, intradermal, patch, or eye test, the Prausnitz-Kustner reaction, or the RAST tests, it must be remembered that exceptions to every rule exist. If you are one of those rare people who react slowly to a test, you need not be discouraged. Your physician can use more than one test. He can search back through your case and family histories for illuminating clues. Remember the proverbial saying, "There's more than one way to skin a cat." This holds true in allergy detection, too. If one method is slow to show results, another can be used until a solution is found. And if all methods fail, the doctor can resort to first-hand observation, usually best accomplished by hospitalization. Even when hospitalization is difficult, he can, when foods are the suspected allergens, continue his analysis by getting a complete list of foods and their amounts eaten daily by the patient.

Removing the cause

After the patient has been examined, tested, and proved to be allergic, treatment to remove the cause begins. If the illness has been traced to an infection, this must be treated or removed.

In cases of serum allergy, the best treatment is the prevention of further exposure to the allergen. Drugs may be used if the immediate symptoms are severe enough. The best remedy, however, is scrupulous avoidance of serums by the patient.

If the allergy is occupational, a number of measures may prevent a recurrence of symptoms. Gloves and long-sleeved shirts or jackets keep the allergen from touching the skin and producing rashes or eczema. Although inhaled allergens are much more difficult to control, masks have been found to be helpful. Further precautions should be taken by workers who, though not allergic themselves, have spouses and children who are. Unwittingly, these workers may bring factory dusts home on their clothing and thus become "carriers" to their families, some of whose members may soon show allergic symptoms. Such cases are not widespread, but when they do occur, they may be extremely puzzling to both the victim and the allergist who is not alerted to this possibility.

The patient who reacts to animal danders must get rid of all cats, dogs, birds, and other household pets, and avoid contact with these animals in the homes of his friends. Pillows stuffed with goose feathers should also be removed, and dacron or rubber pillows substituted.

A person who suffers from a "weather" allergy can apply ointments to his skin if he is sensitive to the sun's rays. Further precautions include wearing gloves, stockings, veils, and long-sleeved garments. Those who are sensitive to heat or cold must avoid all extremes of temperature in order to prevent serious constitutional reactions.

Avoiding serums and animal danders and wearing protective clothing are only preventive measures. Sometimes they work, but most often, they do not. As a result, it becomes necessary in a great many cases to desensitize the individual. Such treatment is administered with great care.

In allergies to heat, desensitizing is accomplished by exposing the patient to higher and higher temperatures for longer and longer periods. Likewise, cold sensitivity is cured by slowly increasing the patient's contact with gradually lower temperatures. This may be accomplished by baths in water of prescribed temperatures. If attempts to desensitize fail, the patient must carefully avoid extreme temperatures. Even if this is impossible, the patient can get temporary relief by using hot or cold applications, according to his condition.

The most encouraging results of desensitization have occurred among persons who are allergic to tree, plant, weed, and grass pollen. By using an extract made from the allergen, many allergists have been able to make their patients either partially or completely immune to the cause of their hay fever or asthma. The most frequently used extracts are ragweed, timothy, plantain, sorrel, oak, birch, poplar, elm, sycamore, beech, cedar, ash, maple, hickory, cocklebur, aster, dahlia, chrysanthemum, and cosmos.

The quickest and most efficient method of using these substances is to find out which pollens are causing the symptoms. These substances are then combined into one extract. In this way, one injection does the work of several. The combination dosage saves the patient the annoyance of separate injections for each of the allergens.

In preparing these mixtures, the allergist considers the pollens to which the individual reacts, the season in which the pollens are present, the intensity and recurrence of symptoms, and the pollen count at the time of the injection. For example, a patient needs a smaller dose during pollination seasons.

As mentioned in "Hay Fever," the injections may be pre-seasonal, co-seasonal, or perennial. The pre-seasonal method establishes the patient's maximum tolerance before the pollination season begins. Weekly injections are given.

The co-seasonal type is used when treatment begins just prior to, or during the season. Small doses are given every day for three days and slowly increased in strength every two, three, or four days.

The perennial treatment consists of injections every four weeks during the winter and as often as necessary during the pollination season.

Of the three types, pre-seasonal treatment usually gives the best results.

Desensitization has been achieved in cases of

allergy to bacteria by making vaccines from sputum, sinus, nasal, or bronchial discharges. This vaccine is injected weekly in increasing amounts until the maximum tolerance has been reached. Then the maximum dose is given every two to four weeks for as long as is necessary. However, if the patient reacts negatively, the injections are either reduced or stopped. This is seldom necessary, and on the whole vaccine treatments are effective against hay fever, asthma, and skin rashes caused by bacteria.

Environmental factors

Important in the treatment of allergy is the patient's environment, which is extremely hard to control. Nevertheless, certain precautionary steps can be taken at home, at work, and at play. Where the climate and the locale affect the patient adversely, some controls can also be established.

At home

At home, dust frequently causes or affects an allergy. For this reason, cleanliness is a necessity. Heavy draperies, furniture, and rugs should be removed and light, smooth-surfaced articles substituted. Many people have found, to their delight, that this substitution not only improved their health but made their homes more cheerful.

Two of the ingredients of house dust in a number of homes are animal dander and animal saliva, both of which may be sensitizers. If the patient shows any reaction to either or both of them, he must remove them from his house. Often people who have sneezing spells accompanied by watering and redness of the eyes own rabbits, cats, dogs, or birds. Consequently, the allergist investigates the possibility of household pets in cases of perennial asthma or hay fever.

Other allergens in the home are insecticides, disinfectants, and washing powders. If some brands are found to be allergens, they should be discarded immedately and new brands tried.

At work

The environmental allergens that are contacted vary, naturally, with the occupations. The chemist or factory worker who handles chemicals in the course of his daily duties may become asthmatic by inhaling certain commercial compounds. He may also experience itching, burning, and sores on the skin from handling these materials. Protective clothing is helpful in these cases. If such protection fails to give relief, the allergist may attempt desensitization. Where this is impossible, the individual may be forced to change his occupation to get away from the allergen.

There are many other cases of sensitivity to substances used at work, such as the druggist or the physician who reacts to the handling of certain medicines, the baker who is sensitive to flour, the dentist who is allergic to novocaine, the cartoonist who gets a rash when he touches inks, and the beautician who cannot tolerate hair dyes.

At play

In our discussion of environmental factors associated with play, we must consider both the child who contacts allergic dust on toys or poison ivy on a picnic, and the adult who is exposed to allergens during occasional leisure hours or on vacation. For example, a person may have trouble only when he takes his annual fishing trip to the Great Lakes area. In this area, we find an important allergen, the scales shed by the caddis fly. Another case is the person who suffers from heat sensitivity on a cruise in the tropics. These cases and thousands of similar ones are, as a rule, easy to diagnose because the symptoms appear suddenly, and during a time when the patient is likely to be most conscious of his surroundings. If the patient cannot be desensitized to the allergen, the physician may suggest a change to resorts or locales which are free from that allergen.

Locale

The subject of locale is just as important to the native of a given area as it is to the vacationer. Proof of this can easily be found by looking through the case histories of the allergic inhabitants of a humid coastal city and comparing them with those of persons living in an area where ragweed is most abundant. We find that a number of cases of allergy among the coastal people are caused by molds which grow well in a warm, moist climate. On the other hand, the people who live in the ragweed area show a predominance of respiratory diseases from that allergen. It is interesting to note that there are many more cases of hay fever and asthma in the United States than in any other country in the world because of the huge amount of ragweed that grows here.

The heavily wooded sections of this country are

sources of tree and plant pollens, and the South and Midwest produce a great number of grass pollens. Whatever the area, the allergist can only prescribe a change of locale if the patient cannot be desensitized. If such a change is impossible, drugs which give temporary relief may be prescribed.

Climate

Climate is, of course, as important as locale, temperature, humidity, and seasonal changes because it makes possible the growth of allergens. The truly unfortunate allergic victim is the one who finds that his city or state, by reason of its climate, is loaded with an allergen or allergens that he can escape only by resettling. Happily, such people are in the minority. However, a great many hay fever and asthma victims who live in moist climates have had relief from their ailments when they moved to drier regions. Resettling is often equally beneficial for persons allergic to molds, and is sometimes used as a last recourse in the fight against stubborn physical allergies. For example, a cold-sensitive patient may lose all his allergic symptoms after having moved to parts of southern California or to Florida.

The allergic individual whose condition is caused by climate does not necessarily have to change his residence permanently. It may be sufficient for him to merely avoid one season in his home city or state. The air may be infested with a certain allergen during one time of the year. During the other three seasons, he can live at home with no discomfort. (See Part II.)

When a change to another climate is impossible, the use of medicines may give temporary relief.

Additional comfort may be obtained by installing air-conditioning in the home and office to filter pollens and dust from the air. If the expense of these units is prohibitive, window ventilators, which are much cheaper, may be used. Or, at no cost at all, the windows in the allergic person's room can be closed while the door is left ajar to provide fresh air from adjoining rooms. Any of these methods will greatly reduce the patient's exposure to pollens and other airborne allergens.

Eat wisely but well

The final topic in our discussion of allergy treatment is diets. When the allergist uses elimination diets to discover specific food allergens, he prescribes a nourishing group of nonallergic foods which the patient can eat safely. The change is achieved with a minimum of discomfort to the sensitized person. Nonessential foods are easily avoided, and a variety of other foods may serve as adequate substitutes for certain nutritious foods.

Restricting the diets of infants and young children is more serious. Where the whey from cow's milk is the allergen, the use of human, goat's or mare's milk is prescribed. However, cow's milk can usually be made safe if it is boiled six hours before a feeding. If evaporated milk is used, it should be boiled ten minutes. Soybean milks are also helpful and do not cause nutritional deficiencies.

If the infant is allergic to the casein in milk, he may be unable to digest this food, cooked or raw. Here, again, the soybean preparations are beneficial. Another substitute is porridge to which the necessary vitamins, minerals, fats, and proteins have been added. In addition, amino acid preparations are good for allergic infants. These preparations have a rather unpleasant taste and odor, making them less desirable for older children and adults whose tastes are more highly developed.

When the allergies are caused by seasonal fruits and vegetables such as tomatoes, corn, asparagus, strawberries, raspberries, peaches, plums, cantaloupe, celery, and watermelons, the infant's diet may only be limited during one season of the year.

People with skin diseases must often avoid those spices and foods which make a meal enjoyable. Pepper, mustard, horse-radish, tabasco, chili sauces, curry, alcohol, tea, and coffee are removed from the diet. These foods affect the blood circulation and thus may aggravate the skin disorder.

If the foods to be eliminated are essential to nourishment, the allergist replaces them with others which contain all the diet essentials. For example, a diet that is free of milk and cheese is apt to lack calcium. To overcome this deficiency, green, leafy vegetables, molasses, and maple syrup are prescribed. Other foods which are rich in calcium are filberts, turnips, and rhubarb.

Meat and fish supply valuable proteins and phosphorus. If they are removed from the diet, nuts and lentils should be substituted. Cereals are beneficial in planning restrictive diets because they produce much-needed energy.

In other cases, a diet low in table salt is followed.

Special attention is also given to keeping the patient's weight normal. There are many nutritious and palatable diets which do just that. Bran is an effective aid in avoiding constipation. A "must" in nearly all diets is the drinking of large amounts of water.

The value of any diet in the treatment of an allergy

depends upon the experience of the allergist who prescribes it and the care with which the patient follows it. If the patient allows himself to become careless, a relapse may occur at any time, and among highly sensitized individuals this may be annoying and sometimes dangerous. The allergist points this out to his patient who, in turn, should tell well-meaning friends and relatives that he is not allowed to eat everything they urge upon him. Occasionally a friend slips into a hospital or sickroom and "treats" the patient to a food forbidden by his physician. Acts of this sort, though understandable, can be extremely detrimental to the patient's recovery.

Sometimes a diet treatment which does not completely exclude a food allergen is tried. In this method, a small amount of the sensitizer is allowed to remain in the diet. The portions are gradually increased until, theoretically, the patient is completely immune. Similar treatment in pollen allergy has been very successful. Unfortunately, the results in food immunization have not been too good, and many of these diets have proved valueless. Therefore, the diet which completely excludes an allergic substance is best in treating food allergy, provided adequate precautions are taken to prevent vitamin and mineral deficiencies.

Look to the future

"A stitch in time saves nine" is an old proverb that applies to the allergist's field. An allergist is concerned not only with cures but also with prevention and reduction of allergic attacks. Preventive treatments for "nonallergic" and allergic individuals vary. Considered in the "nonallergic" group are those persons whose family histories show no cases of allergy. In addition to the immense number of patients with hereditary tendencies toward allergies, many persons with no apparent family history of asthma, hay fever, skin rashes, digestive or cardio-vascular symptoms, or sinusitis may suffer from allergic reactions. In such cases, the allergy is acquired through exposure to an allergen.

Preventive measures for the nonallergic

High on the list of preventive measures is cleanliness. Factory workers and chemists who handle dyes, drugs, and chemicals should wash their hands often. Frequent bathing is always helpful in preventing allergy and in maintaining general good health.

Another preventive measure is to avoid taking drugs. The discovery and increased popularity of antibiotics have caused many people to take them for every minor ailment. They are unaware of the dangerous reactions that may occur when allergic sensitivity is present. Too often, people take drugs such as aspirin and sleeping pills without consulting their physician. Anyone who uses these "self treatments" has only himself to blame for the discomforts that follow.

Another cause of allergy is the large number of infections which remain untreated. Everyone agrees that the sooner an unhealthy condition is treated, the greater are the possibilities for recovery. Yet, an unbelievably large number of people who give lip service to this common theory let their own bodily ailments run a chronic course. In medical literature, innumerable cases of allergy caused by bacteria and other microorganisms have been found. Unless these infections receive immediate attention, there is great danger of both allergic reactions, and irreparable degeneration of the tissues involved and consequent partial or total disability.

Chronic infections are frequently present for many years before an allergy develops, but patients of all ages are susceptible to sensitization from bacteria and other infectious agents. Many persons begin to suffer from asthma around the age of forty.

Because of hereditary sensitivity, the second group of allergic people may react to all known allergens. If one parent is allergic, the child is likely to develop an allergy; if both parents are subject to any of the various allergies, there is a much greater possibility that their child will be allergic, and that it will appear at an earlier age. The child's symptoms need not be identical to those of his parents. For example, the mother may have a skin rash from cosmetics, the father asthma from ragweed pollen, and the child digestive irregularities from shellfish.

Because of the enormous number of allergens and because they can produce symptoms in any part of the body, there is no general treatment. Instead, the allergist must seek to remove as many sensitizers as possible from the patient's daily life. A number of beneficial measures can be taken without altering the patient's normal routine.

Since food is one of the first substances to which an infant is exposed, certain precautions in feeding should be taken. A baby who has either one or two allergic parents should receive special attention when fed protein foods. All cow's milk should be dried, condensed, or boiled. Raw vegetables, raw fruits, and their juices should be given in small amounts. The mother or nurse should avoid giving the infant an excessive amount of food of any type.

By using the Prausnitz-Kustner method of testing, the allergist is often able to predict the foods to which the child will react negatively in later life. Research has shown that allergies are sometimes discovered by this method before the young patient has been exposed to them. It is like gazing into a scientific crystal ball, since the tests provide an accurate guide in planning future treatment.

In preventing drug allergy, the procedure with the hereditary group is much the same as with the non-hereditary group. In the hereditary group, even greater care is required in the use of antibiotics, sulfonamides, quinine, aspirin, iodine, and serums, whether taken by injection or by mouth.

Cleanliness can prevent many reactions to pollen, dust, and animal allergens. All furniture, draperies, floors, and bedding should be kept spotless since accumulation of dust increases the possibility of sensitization. Avoid exposure to animal danders or feathers. Cats, dogs, canaries, and other household pets should be removed from the home.

Cosmetics should only be used in moderation. Toiletries which contain rice flour or orris-root should not be used.

Inhalation of any large amount of ant, roach, or other insecticide powders should be carefully avoided. These substances are widely used, frequently in a careless manner. They are a threat not only to the person who is apt to become allergic, but to infants and babies who may get the insecticide on their fingers and swallow it.

Without adequate treatment, little can be done to

prevent sensitivity to pollen except to try to avoid the allergen. Pollen charts can be secured from an allergist. He is also able to suggest areas where the air is comparatively free of these allergens. A summer vacation in locales where the pollen count is extremely high is a foolish risk. The higher the count, the greater the probability of symptoms.

Bacteria, as well as other infectious agents, may be a dangerous allergen. Sinusitis, particularly, may be the forerunner of a multitude of both allergic and nonallergic diseases.

The infectious agents of many childhood ailments such as measles, mumps, chicken pox, and diphtheria may become sensitizers. Where possible, foci of infection should be removed. In any case, immediate treatment is essential.

Prevention of infection is a good way to avoid future allergies. Simple measures such as adequate rest and exercise, well-planned meals, correct weight, fresh air, sunshine, and complete avoidance of contact with persons who have infectious or contagious diseases contribute immeasurably to the patient's continued health.

Chapter XIII
NEW FRONTIERS

New biochemical tools are helping scientists forge ahead in knowledge in the field of allergy. How can the development of allergic reactions be prevented? The answer may lie in preventing the production of the antibody IgE. Immunologists are trying to find the answers.

But much practical work of more immediate value is being done, too. A network of asthma and allergic disease centers has been established throughout the country by the National Institute of Allergy and Infectious Diseases (NIAID). Network scientists work closely with clinical allergists to expand knowledge of allergic disease.

Until allergy can be prevented, treatment of allergic symptoms is going through improvements and refinements. One method is to use only the *part* of the allergen responsible for its allergy-causing activity in desensitizing injections. Antigens E, K,

Ra3, and Ra5 have already been isolated from ragweed. Being tested in animals, these fractions will be used in clinical investigations on people.

Study is also going ahead on modifying the allergens used in desensitization. "Allergoids" have been prepared from rye grass or mixed grass pollen extracts treated with formaldehyde. Allergoids appear to help produce protective antibodies without causing as much of an allergic reaction as untreated extracts.

Although persons with allergies still have many problems, their future looks markedly brighter.

PART II

Chapter XIV
HINTS ABOUT THE HOME

General precautions

Every day more nonallergenic products are being developed for the home. Some are excellent, but be sure to read all the fine print before you buy. Or consult a consumer protection group. In general, plant and animal products should be eliminated and synthetics substituted (e.g. Dacron). If you are in doubt about whether to use a particular product, get in touch with:

Allergy-Free Products for the Home
1162 West Lynn
Springfield, MO 65802

Allergy-Free Products for the Home
224 Livingstone Street
Brooklyn, NY 11201

Allergen-Proof Encasings
1450 East 363rd Street
Eastlake, OH 44094

If dust bothers you, cover your mouth and nose with several layers of damp gauze before you clean, and use a damp cloth for dusting. Keep away from dusty attics, storerooms, etc.

Avoid smoke as well as irritating odors from stoves, lamps, paints, tobacco, camphor, and tar.

Do not keep pets unless tested specifically for them.

Get someone else to spray with an insecticide.

Keep the bedroom closed off from the rest of the house and be sure to use nonallergenic pillows and mattress covers.

How to obtain a dust sample

If this is what your allergist needs, here is an easy way to do it.

Remove the cloth bag from your vacuum cleaner. Turn on the machine for a minute or two to free the mechanism from present dust. Tie a piece of muslin on the machine in the place of the cloth bag. Then operate it directly or by one of its attachments. Try to collect a tablespoon of dust from the mattress, pillows, and linen of the patient's bed. Remove the cloth, fold and label it. Then, tie another clean piece of muslin in its place, and test the living room rug. In the same way, you can obtain samples from all of the rugs, from the automobile, and any other likely source of dust in the home or working environment.

Air-conditioning

If your allergist suggests air-conditioning or an air filter to be used in the home, you may rent one and use it in the bedroom or a closed room for a month or two to determine the extent of relief. Insofar as size, one with an air flow that is sufficient to provide an air exchange in the room five or six times per hour is preferable. The size of the room in cubic feet also makes a difference. A small room takes a small unit. The use of an activated charcoal filter effectively lessens the output of ozone produced by the operation of an electrostatic precipitator. The unit must be cleaned often, and the directions given by the manufacturer should be followed.

When buying, you should be wary of any exaggerated sales claims for appliances that are not capable of real air purification. Even ordinary vacuum cleaners have been promoted for preventing or treating respiratory ailments. Effective air purification equipment is available but is more costly than the small units incapable of removing dust and pollen. Although air-treatment devices are being sold as "negative ion generators," it has not been established that negative ions are of any value for preventing or treating disease.

Preventing mildew

Fresh air, sun, and electric bulbs are the enemies of mildew, a potent allergen. Leave closet (including the linen closet) doors and dresser drawers open now and then for plenty of ventilation. Use an electric fan in places that cannot be aired. Be sure to dry dirty clothes before you put them in the hamper. Clean or wash clothing before you store it. Wash laundry or sizing out of garments before storing, and expose garments stored in bags to sun and air from time to time. By replacing 20 percent or more of the regular pigment with zinc oxide, a mildew-resistant paint may be made.

Chapter XV

HINTS ABOUT THE OUTDOORS

What to do when the air is polluted

The asthmatic inevitably has more symptoms—coughing, wheezing, and dyspnea—during an episode of air pollution than at other times. He will also, along with many others, have burning sensations in his throat and eyes.

If you have these symptoms severely or persistently, it is best to consult your physician. There are, however, things you can do to help yourself.

(1) Do not engage in unnecessary physical activity.

(2) Do not smoke or go into smoke-filled rooms.

(3) Stay away from dusts and other irritants such as hair spray, insect spray, exhaust fumes, or any kind of smoke.

161

(4) Stay away from those with colds and respiratory infection.

(5) Stay indoors in a clear environment with closed windows. Air-conditioning as well as charcoal filters and electrostatic precipitators may be helpful.

(6) Should the pollution persist or worsen, it might be best to leave the area.

Major pollutants include:

Total suspended particulates. These are solid and liquid particles in the atmosphere, including dust, smoke mists, fumes, and sprays from many sources.

Sulfur dioxide. A heavy, pungent, colorless gas formed from the combustion of coal and oil.

Carbon monoxide. An invisible, odorless, poisonous gas, mainly derived from incomplete combustion of carbon fuels and industrial processes involving carbonaceous material. More than 50 percent comes from motor vehicles.

Ozone (as O_3). Pungent, colorless, toxic gas, a component of photochemical fog.

Nitrogen dioxide. Brown, toxic gas formed from fuel combustion. It may be associated with ozone production under certain conditions.

Climate

Occasionally an allergic patient and his allergist decide that a change of climate might be best. In such cases, the physician will describe in detail the type of climate that would best suit the patient. If you need it, you can obtain information on where such climates can be found from the National Climatic Center, Federal Building, Asheville, North Carolina 28801.

In addition, there are pollen guides available which show areas which have, or do not have, significant amounts of certain pollens. Medical societies or local chambers of commerce also may be sources of information about allergens in proposed areas.

For the insect-sting sensitive who love the outdoors

The hiker, golfer, or picnicker who knows he is allergic to bee or other insect stings should not count on finding a physician or hospital in the wilderness or right next to a golf course.

If you are one of these people, ask your physician about a kit that contains a tourniquet, an oral antihistamine, and an injectable epinephrine in a prefilled syringe. One such kit is the Ana-Kit (R) made by Hollister-Stier Laboratories. Laws vary in different states and sometimes a patient is not allowed any such injectable. In such cases, inhalable or sublingual epinephrine may be used.

Before going into insect country, make sure that you are *adequately* protected.

Chapter XVI

HINTS ABOUT DRUGS AND DIETS

Drugs

One of the most important "rules" for the allergic person to follow is to check out any drug whatsoever with the physician before taking it. Sometimes there is a component in an over-the-counter medicine which can cause trouble, such as yeast in a vitamin tablet.

Common drug allergens are:

aspirin
penicillin
sulfonamides
antituberculous drugs
nitrofurans
barbiturates

anticonvulsants
local anesthetics
phenolphthalein
quinine and quinidine
iodides and bromides
organ extracts (ACTH, insulin)
heavy metals
sera and vaccines
tranquilizers
antithyroid drugs
aminopyrine

Elimination diet

For persons suspected of being allergic to food, the following method of elimination diet is widely used.

Tested first is the most consumed group of foods—which contains a large amount of protein—such as meats, milk, egg, wheat, rice, rye, oats, chicken, pork, lamb, beef, codfish, halibut, tea, coffee, chocolate, mustard, coconut, and peanuts.

The second series, which contains a lesser amount of protein, includes such fruits and vegetables as oranges, grapefruit, bananas, peaches, prunes, apples, strawberries, onions, potatoes, carrots, celery, cabbage, corn, spinach, cucumber, lima beans, peas, and tomatoes.

In the third series are lemons, apricots, cantaloupes, dates, figs, grapes, pineapple, pears, honeydew melon, lettuce, cauliflower, green peas, parsley, soya beans, sweet potatoes, turnips, pecans, and walnuts.

Remember, each of the three series may be varied or rearranged by the individual physician. There is no set rule for the order or for the kind of food tested.

Cooking means substituting

In a day when a substitute may be found for almost any type of food, a special diet for the allergic person does not pose the problems it once did.

Rice flour and corn starch are good substitutes for wheat flour. There is also rye flour, potato starch, pure buckwheat, and barley flour. Health food stores are apt to carry these. There are several milk and cream substitutes often used in coffee. Almost any moderately skilled cook can have a good time seeing what ingenuity and substituting will do.

For someone who is allergic to wheat and milk, try some rice waffles:

2 cups rice flour
2 cups cream substitute
4 tablespoons melted margarine
½ teaspoon salt
4 teaspoons baking powder
2 eggs, separated

Mix all ingredients except egg whites together. Beat egg whites until stiff and fold them in. Cook on your waffle iron until brown and crisp. This recipe serves four people.

Even for cooks who are not adventurous, there are plenty of recipes for allergic people.

Some of the recipes listed below are free. Write for further details.

Name of diet	*Name of company putting out the diet*
Baking for People with Food Allergies	Superintendent of Documents

	U.S. Government Printing Office Washington, DC 20402
Recipes for the Allergic Individual	Kannengiesser & Company 76 Ninth Avenue New York, NY 10011
Cooking with Imagination for Special Diets	Grocery Store Products Company West Chester, PA 19380
Fast and Fancy Desserts from Richwhip (Milk Substitute)	Rich Products Corporation 1145 Niagara Street Buffalo, NY 14213
Diets Unlimited for Limited Diets	Allergy Information Association 3 Powburn Place Weston 627, Ontario, Canada
125 Great Recipes for Allergy Diets	*Good Housekeeping* 969 Eighth Avenue New York, NY 10019
Allergy Recipes from the Blue Flame Kitchen	Metropolitan Utilities District 1723 Harney Street Omaha, NE 68102
Allergy Recipes	The American Dietetic Association 620 North Michigan Avenue Chicago, IL 60611
Good Eating for the Milk-Sensitive Person	Ross Laboratories 625 Cleveland Avenue Columbus, OH 43216

Easy Appealing Recipes (Milk-Free Diets)	Mead Johnson Laboratories Department 852 Evansville, IN 47721
Allergy Diets	Ralston Purina Company Nutrition Service Checkerboard Square St. Louis, MO 63199

In addition, milk-free, egg-free, wheat-free, and gluten-free products many be obtained from:

Beech-Nut Baby Foods
605 Third Avenue
New York, NY 10016

General Mills
9200 Wayzata Boulevard
Minneapolis, MI 55440

Ener-G-Foods
1526 Utah Avenue South
Seattle, WA 98123